"I've been in home he
been the greatest lear

"I learned about making intangible things become tangible. One of the things I need to do right away is classify my A, B, and C referrals and follow up on them."

**— Hershey Glenn, Director of Services,
NHC Homecare, Tennessee**

"I've learned a ton and plan on implementing a lot of what I've learned in my offices with my staff. I'm looking forward to having our numbers go up with these great ideas. I highly recommend it to anyone who is interested in boosting their numbers."

**— Lisa Miller, Owner,
A Trinity Valley Home Health and Therapy Services, Texas**

"Lots of wonderful information and tools available. I just wish I had gotten involved sooner."

**— Bob Zangas,
All Metro Health Care, Missouri**

"I'm very excited to implement a lot of the objectives I've learned on how to get referrals and how to maintain them and the follow-up I need to do to run my business."

**— Melissa Rinch, Administrator,
NHC Homecare, Florida**

"So many tools I could use on a daily and weekly basis. Using the sales tools, I can create a solid plan of action for my sales calls. Plus, I got a ton of marketing ideas. It's great."

**— Stacy Montgomery, Account Executive,
Guardian Home Care, Tennessee**

"I'm a very active marketer but he has helped me to narrow my focus down. I really want to build my orthopedic program and he gave me some ideas about hospitalists and most of all that I'm not closing the deal on some of the calls, so I'm going to refocus; I'm going to get my team activated. We're going to spread out and we're going to hit it."

— Julie Coates, Administrator,
NHC Homecare, South Carolina

"I'm very excited about all of the ideas that I've learned. I would highly recommend it for anyone wanting to increase referrals and boost employee morale."

— Angie Roberts, Director of Nursing,
A Trinity Valley Home Health and Therapy Services, Texas

"Field-tested, proven and practical approaches that will promote and grow your home care business. Adam knows home care and these innovative ideas really work."

— Michael Pohanka, President,
Community Care Services, Ontario

"I've been a care coordinator now for five years and I've gotten to the point in my marketing where I reached a plateau — bringing in referrals here and there but nothing tremendous. But now, with these materials, it's opened my eyes to a whole new level of marketing that I've never known about. I promise, you will be amazed."

— Christopher Veith, Care Coordinator,
Ever Caring Home Health Care, Illinois

FREE FREE

Critique Certificate

This certificate entitles bearer to submit any single printed piece, brochure, direct-mail piece, advertisement, website or similar promotional material by mail or fax for critique by TAG Home Care Marketing.

Name:________________________________

Company:________________________________

Agency Type: ❑ Home Health ❑ Private Duty ❑ Hospice ❑ Other:____________

Address:________________________________

City:________________ State:________ Zip:________

Tel:________________ Fax:________________

E-mail:________________________________

Date Issued:________________

TOTAL VALUE: $100

Send Certificate and promotional material to:

TAG Home Care Marketing
115 Southeast Parkway Court
Franklin, TN 37064
FAX: 1–866–232–6470

Terms & Conditions: Certificate expires 12 months from date of issue. Please allow 3 to 4 weeks for response from TAG Home Care Marketing. Consultation given by mail only. Actual finished materials or "rough sketch" and copy for planned material may be submitted. Coupon redeemable only for listed services. Additional consulting may be submitted for review by TAG Home Care Marketing. Any piece submitted with critique coupons may be published in any TAG Home Care Marketing authored/edited publications, as examples. Also, submitted materials will not be returned.

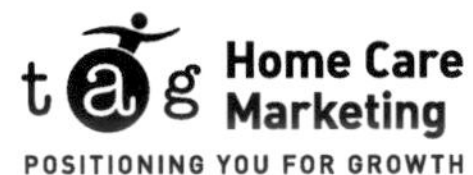

866–232–6477

FREE www.theadamgrp.com FREE

REVISED SECOND EDITION

48 PROVEN STEPS

To Successfully Market Your HOME CARE SERVICES

Home Health ■ Hospice ■ Private Duty

Adam D. Bishop, MBA

Judith A. Bishop, RN

Library of Congress Control Number: 2001130576

Published by:
TAG Publishing
115 Southeast Parkway Ct.
Franklin, Tennessee 37064
Tel: 615-794-1436
Fax: 615-791-5935

Cover Design: G. Seth West
Inside Design and Layout: Miranda Fuller
Edited by: Kathryn Knight

DISCLAIMER AND/OR LEGAL NOTICES:

While all attempts have been made to verify information provided in this book, neither the Authors nor the Publisher assumes any responsibility for errors, insurances or omissions. Any slights of people or organizations are unintentional. If advice concerning legal or related matters is needed, the services of a qualified professional should be sought. This book is not intended for use as a source of legal or accounting advice. Also, some suggestions made in this book concerning marketing, sales etc., may have inadvertently introduced practices deemed unlawful in certain states and municipalities. Any references to any persons or businesses, whether living or dead, existing or defunct, is purely coincidental.

PRINTED IN THE UNITED STATES OF AMERICA

Home Care Professional

We hope this book will assist you and your staff by providing a framework upon which to build the kind of advertising, publicity and marketing that will help your Home Care Company achieve profitable and successful growth.

The idea of marketing Home Care services makes many Home Care professionals and entrepreneurs uncomfortable. Because of the cost-based reimbursement and regulatory issues regarding the disallowance of marketing costs, many home health care managers have not had the experience of marketing their business effectively.

However, there has never been a better time to re-evaluate old strategies and develop creative ways to expand, diversify, and increase your company's revenues and profitability. *Your future depends on developing methods of getting and keeping clients.*

This book presents numerous ideas, anecdotes, and innovative marketing techniques that Home Care companies have used to make their businesses prosper. Innovative thinking is often lacking in the big agencies and corporations that have the most money to spend. Therefore, the sources for many of the ideas in this book have been small to medium size Home Care companies that have had limited money and resources — but plenty of good ideas that have worked!

Several of the ideas and suggestions in this book may have already occurred to you. You may have tried some with varying degrees of success. Others may be completely new to you and may appear to be a little crazy but they frequently do work.

After spending twenty-five years working in Home Health Care, starting Home Care businesses, and helping to build their successful growth, we know how challenging it is to grow a Home Care business while not compromising professional integrity. We have also experienced first hand the challenges that face caregivers and grown children when arranging and overseeing services for parents and loved ones.

If even *one* of the ideas in this book helps to stimulate your own creative ideas, then it will have been a worthwhile investment of your time and money.

Have fun and good luck.

Adam D. Bishop

Juana C. Bishop

TABLE OF CONTENTS

PART 3
Marketing Does Not End After The Ads Run...

INTRODUCTION

Health care delivery has undergone dramatic changes in recent years. New diagnostic technologies, new drugs, new surgical methods, and new ideas about treatment have all contributed to shorter hospital stays for many patients.

Releasing recovering people from hospitals shifts the costs and responsibility of patient care elsewhere. Relatives and friends of the patient will provide some of this care free. Some will be purchased from private providers of Home Care services.

This is an important driving force behind the increased growth in the Home Care Industry. This industry — particularly private pay home health care — will continue to expand and grow for decades.

It is a fact that older people today have more disposable income than younger people, and they are willing to pay to get what they want, when they want it. The huge wave of aging baby-boomers will be as demanding when it comes to health care as they are when they buy any product or service.

How will your Home Care business stand out from the crowd to attract these clients? How will you compete in the future competitive marketplace as new Home Care businesses spring up to meet the demand?

You will set agency goals.

This sounds easy, but many agencies don't have a clue on where they are going. These goals will be general *and* specific — shared with your entire team.

You will conduct research.

You will gather information about your industry and your competition — their strengths and weaknesses and the strategies that they are using. You will also need to recognize the opportunities and threats of your industry.

You will identify your target market.

Just knowing the demographics of your market is not sufficient. You'll need to account for your audiences' lifestyles and needs, where they work, what factors influence their decisions — and determine how best to reach them.

You will define your image and your brand.

Where specifically do you fit in your market? What position will profit you the most and best fit with your style of service and goals?

You will determine your marketing methods.

Once all the planning groundwork is in place, you will choose the most effective and efficient marketing methods to communicate your message to your audience.

In short, you will market your company.

And this manual will help you immeasurably in understanding, planning, and developing your particular marketing strategy and materials.

PART 1

Laying the Groundwork

CHAPTER ONE

Work On Your Business, *Not In Your Business*

Drive thy business or it will drive thee.

— Benjamin Franklin

What does this mean? Simply, don't let your business own you.

Are you spending most of your time personally providing nursing services services to clients, scheduling visits, and managing employees? Then you are working *in* your business.

Are you spending most of your time developing a marketing plan, researching new opportunities both internally and externally for your agency, expanding your services, and looking into new niches to target? Then you are working *on* your business.

Most agency owners work in their businesses. This isn't necessarily bad, especially for a small start-up agency. However, if you continue to work *in* your business and not *on* your business, growth and success will be minimal — if at all.

There is an old joke about the government bureaucrat descending on the small business owner. He says: "We've received a report that you have some poor fellow working here 18 hours a day, seven days a week, for nothing but room, board, meals, all the tobacco he can smoke and all the liquor he can drink. Is this true?" "Yes I'm afraid it is," admits the owner. "And I'm sorry to say, you're looking at him." Don't let this be you!

You need to be able to step outside of the box and look at the big picture of your business. You are the captain of the ship. Therefore, you must have a clear plan and view of your direction. If you don't, no one else will — and you will end up in a disaster.

As your agency grows, you should work less and less in your business. Delegate all your low value tasks. Reduce your company's dependence on *you* as a day-to-day co-worker. Make it a priority to work more and more on your business.

You can't delegate the task of working on your business to someone else. You have to do it!

If you want to work in a business, I recommend that you get a job in somebody else's agency! But don't go to work in your own; because while you're working, while you're answering telephones, while you're making nursing visits, while you're scheduling your nurses, and while you are doing other things, there is something much more important that *isn't getting done.* It's the work you're not doing — the strategic planning, the entrepreneurial work — which will lead your agency forward, and provide you with more free time and a higher level of financial success.

How to work on your business and not in your business

According to Michael E. Gerber, author of *The E Myth*, "Business Format Franchises have reported a success rate of 95 percent in contrast to the 50 plus percent failure rate of new, independently owned businesses. Where 80 percent of all businesses fail in the first five years, 75 percent of all Business Format Franchises succeed!" Gerber argues that the reason for that success is the Franchise Prototype. The primary reason why the Franchise Prototype is so successful is that it runs on a *system*. The system integrates all the components required to make the franchise work. It transforms the business into a well-run machine, everything working together in tandem toward a realized objective.

- The system runs the business.
- The people run the system.

A system works for a franchise — and it will work for your Home Care company, but only if it is thought out, planned, tested, and monitored. *Only if someone is there working on the business.*

I recommend that your Number One Step toward running a successful, profitable Home Care business be to work on your business rather than in your business. This must become the main focus of your daily activity, the prime motivator for everything you do from this moment forward.

Start believing that your agency is the prototype — or will be the prototype — for 100 more just like it. In other words, pretend that you are going to franchise your agency.

According to Gerber, you must follow these rules when developing systems in your agency:

1. Your franchise model must provide consistent value to your clients, employees, suppliers, and lenders — beyond what they expect.

2. People with the lowest possible level of skill will operate your model, because if your model *depends* on highly skilled people, it's going to be impossible to replicate. You need to think about how you can create a systems-dependent business rather than a people dependent business.

   Note: Good employees — especially in the health care industry — *are* crucial. Nothing will replace professional, capable staff members. However, you want your systems set up so that those great employees you have *can* perform their tasks — more efficiently, more confidently.

3. Your model must stand out as a place of impeccable order. An agency that looks orderly says to your client that your people know what they are doing.

4. All of the work in your model must be documented in Operations Manuals. Documentation provides your people with the structure they need and a written account of how to get the job done in the most efficient and effective way.

5. Your model must provide a uniformly predictable service to the client.

6. Your model must utilize a uniform color, dress, and facilities color. Believe it or not, having a professional-looking image will motivate people to choose you over another agency. Your marketing materials, clothes, cars, invoices, signs, displays should all have a cohesive look with a recognizable continuity about them.

If your business is to provide security, freedom and wealth, you should be working at weaning the business from dependence on you and creating dependence on systems.

Set up systems in your agency. Make it systems-dependent, not people-dependent. This will allow you to work less and less in and more and more on your business. You'll receive rewards you never thought possible.

CHAPTER TWO

Think Marketing

Build a better mousetrap and the world will beat a path to your door.

—Ralph Waldo Emerson

That may have been true then... but it's not true now. No one will come. You have to package and promote that mousetrap. Then they will come.

—Charles Gillette

Why Market Your Services?

Because you must in order to compete, thrive and grow.

Marketing is absolutely critical in improving the odds that your company will be able to increase revenue and thrive in the competitive environment.

Marketing Home Care services carries unique challenges — however, it is one aspect of running your business that you need to understand and implement in order to survive.

Under the cost-reimbursed model for Medicare-covered Home Care services, agencies in the past were excluded from being reimbursed for any costs related to "marketing." Companies who were creative — who explored methods of promotion under the label of Community Education — often had these costs challenged by intermediaries and then these costs were often disallowed.

Some companies, who were able to use cash flow generated from non-Medicare services, simply did not attempt to market Medicare-covered services and concentrated their marketing dollars on the promotion of private pay and staffing services.

Now, with the implementation of the Balanced Budget Act and, more recently, the Prospective Pay reimbursement, many Home Care companies have experienced rapid decline in their patient census and revenue.

Companies that have *survived* the last five years are now forced to find ways to grow, diversify and differentiate themselves from the competition. The severe labor shortage and declining availability of nurses and other paraprofessionals have created additional challenges for Home Care operators. Finding creative ways to recruit and retain staff is yet another challenge facing Home Care companies.

The Home Care industry is made up of thousands of small companies and very few large national chains. This provides potential Home Care clients and referral sources with many companies to choose from. Therefore, it is imperative that companies develop specific strategies and invest in marketing programs *now* to retain their existing business and increase referrals.

Ten Truths About Marketing

1. **The Market is constantly changing.**
   You must get your message out to prospective clients, referral sources and the public. It must be clear, consistent, and you must do it continuously.

2. **People forget — fast.**
   Your company's name must be in the client's mind when the client recognizes a need for Home Care services.

3. **Your competition isn't quitting.**
   The market is becoming more competitive. If you don't take care of your clients with marketing, your competition will.

4. **Marketing strengthens your identity and develops a brand name awareness.**
   It is human nature to choose what is most familiar.

5. **Marketing is essential for survival and growth.**
   You have to market your company if you expect to grow and retain market share.

6. **Marketing enables you to hold onto your old clients.**
   An agency's best source of new clients is previously satisfied clients.

7. **Marketing maintains morale.**
   Advertisements can be motivational reminders to the agency's employees of their image and reputation.

8. **Marketing gives you an advantage.**
   Positioning yourself solidly in the market gives you an edge over competitors who have ceased marketing, or have never marketed.

9. **Marketing allows your business to continue operating.** Marketing helps your agency by communicating the benefits your services provide to clients and prospective clients.

10. **You have invested time and money that you stand to lose.** Once you initiate your marketing plan, do not abandon the plan when you don't see immediate results. Instead, evaluate your plan's effectiveness by monitoring results. Unless you are planning to go out of business, do not cease marketing completely.

CHAPTER THREE

Understand Why Companies Fail

Never rest on your oars as a boss. If you do, the whole company starts sinking.

—Lee J. Iacocca

There are five main reasons why companies fail.

1. **They are conservative and rarely try anything new.**
   They stand by and wonder why they are losing clients and market share.

2. **They tend to only go "half-way."**
   They initiate or imitate but don't follow up, analyze, modify, or complete their plans. Lots of companies get great ideas for new services or pay consultants to advise them on how to increase their market share — then sit back and wait for it to happen.

3. **They aren't consistent.**
   For anything to really work you have to work at it continually and consistently.

4. **They don't have a plan.**
   A company has to have a plan. Without a plan you cannot expect your employees to follow a course of action — and there is no way to evaluate whether that course is leading where you want to go.

5. **They procrastinate.**
   Companies have to make the commitment to follow through on plans. Even if you have to modify or completely change the plan, it is better to do something than to sit still and do nothing.

CHAPTER FOUR

Know What Your Clients and Referral Sources Want — *and Need.*

The formula for success in a service business: Find out what people want and give them more of it and find out what they don't want, and give them less of it.

—Judith A. Bishop

In order for you to market to clients who require Home Care services, you need a very clear idea of their wants, needs, expectations — and dislikes.

Most Home Care clients are senior citizens. Therefore, be keenly aware that an older population is more demanding and more knowledgeable about the products and services it needs, and is less willing to tolerate poor services.

Clients want to know they can trust their Home Care provider, not only with their health and/or housekeeping but also with their personal space. The Home Care company will become a part of that home.

Private pay clients want value for their expenditure — and they want to see that value demonstrated.

All clients, private pay or Medicare-covered, want attentive, professional, quality care — *from care providers who truly do care.*

At the same time, most clients are frightened and uneasy about choosing services. It is less risky for them to do nothing than to make the wrong choice. It may be the first time they have ever had to rely on anyone other than a family member to provide them assistance.

Knowing what makes your client "tick" will enable you to reach out and address that need or fear. For instance, because you know that older clients prefer to make an informed choice, you might be wise to offer to have one of your staff make an introductory "house call" to discuss your company. Once they can put a face to your company, they will become more comfortable and you can begin to build a trust/bond.

Referral Sources

It is also important to understand what features and benefits will influence referral sources.

I have outlined some of the features and benefits these various groups have identified as being critical in the selection of a Home Care company. You may have additional ideas to add, but these will provide you with some ideas to think about.

When referring clients to a Home Care company, what factors do you consider?

Physicians responded:

- A competent, qualified staff
- Length of time in business
- Experience in caring for specific needs of their patients
- Provision of appropriate amount and level of care
- Follow-up and communication
- Execution of prescribed treatment and medication orders

Physicians are under pressure from hospitals and long-term care facilities to discharge patients as soon as possible. Doctors are concerned about malpractice suits as a result of early or premature discharges. Home Care agency staff must provide physicians and/or medical directors with evidence that they possess the clinical knowledge and experience to carry out their duties.

Physicians and medical directors appreciate one-on-one verbal communication. Knowing this tells you how to market best to this referral source. Group discussions, writing letters, sending newsletters, etc., may be useful, but will never replace the effectiveness of one-on-one contact.

Discharge Planners/Case Managers responded:

- All of the above plus:
- Quick response and professionalism
- Availability of staff
- Supervision of care

Case managers are interested in finding ways to do more for patients using fewer resources. Home Care agencies should present ways to deliver care that will be efficient and cost effective. They get better results when they address the needs of the case manager by packaging services. They appreciate and remember those Home Care providers who communicate often and keep them updated on their clients' progress.

Trust Officers and Lawyers responded:

- All of the above plus:
- Financial stability of the Home Care agency
- Careful screening of employees — are they bonded and insured and supervised
- Policies in place regarding handling of a client's money
- Invoices — timely and accurate

Family Members and Friends responded:

- All of the above plus:
- Frequent caring communication regarding the status and needs of their loved one
- Trust
- A clear sense that caregivers are compassionate and caring

WHO INFLUENCES HOME CARE BUYING DECISIONS

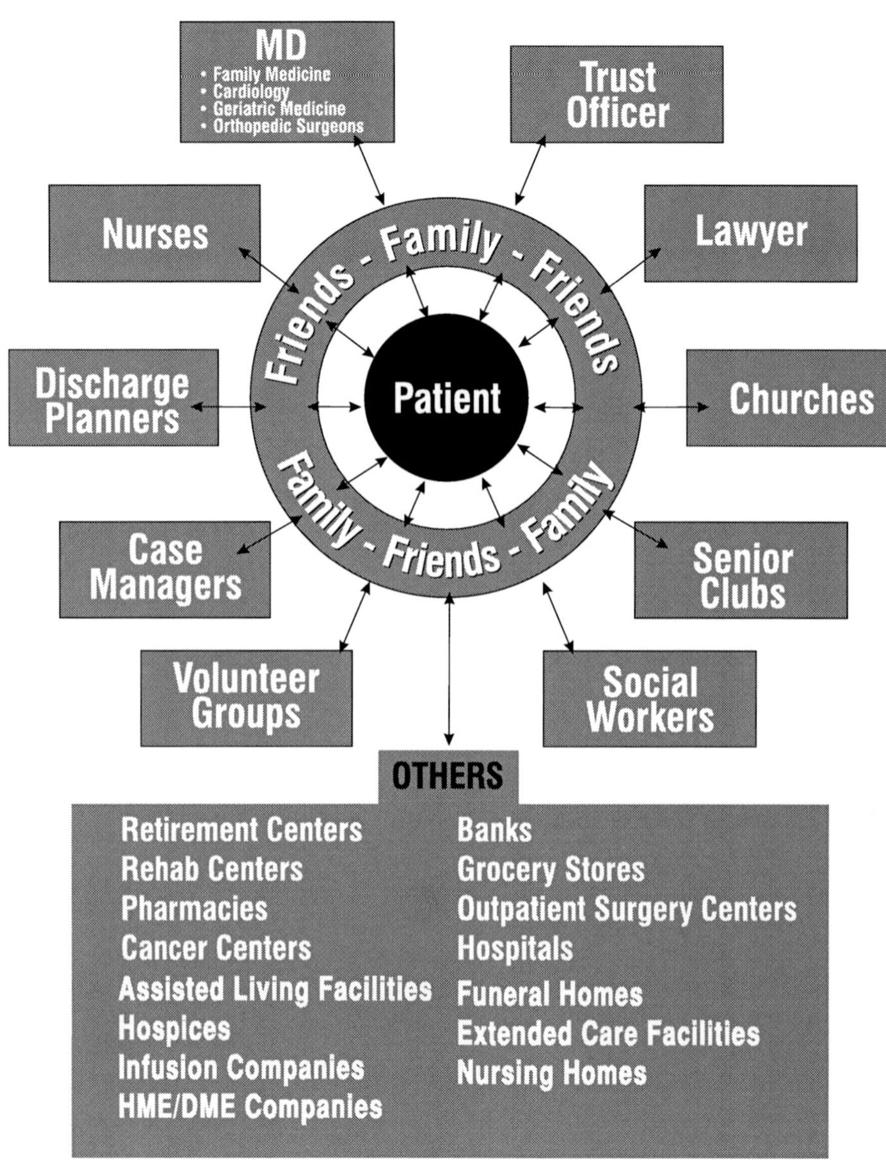

CHAPTER FIVE

Know Which Market Factors Affect Your Business

Keep in mind that you can't control your own future. Your destiny is not in your hands; it is in the hands of the irrational consumer and society. The changes in their needs, desires, and demands will tell you where you must go. All this means that managers must themselves feel the pulse of change on a daily, continuous basis...They should have intense curiosity, observe events, analyze trends, seek the clue of change, and translate those clues into opportunities.

— Michael J. Kami

Every agency operates within an ever-changing network of opportunities and threats — from the external environment, the political/legal arena, and from internal strengths and weaknesses.

Four Market Forces

Four overall — or macro — market-environmental forces affect all agencies: Political/Legal, Economic, Technological, and Social. These forces in general are constantly changing and can not be controlled by the agency directly. Thus, whoever can enable their agency to operate effectively within environmental threats by capitalizing on the opportunity provided by the environment will be the leader in the marketplace.

1. **Political/Legal Forces** include legislation and court judgments, as well as decisions by various commissions and agencies at every level of government, tax laws, consumer industry regulations, and laws on hiring, firing, promotion, and wage or price controls.

2. **Economic Forces** can also have an effect on your business operation. For example, consider the increases or decreases in gross domestic product and the rising or falling of interest rates and inflation. These changes can present both opportunities and threats to your agency.

   Three Economic forces will have the most impact on your business:

   A. *Unemployment Rates and Disposable Personal Income*
   An increase in Gross Domestic Product (GDP) produces a healthy economy, which leads to increased demand for outputs and increased consumer expenditures. This provides great opportunities for both new and established agencies. Decreased GDP could lead to reduced consumer spending. The smart business will watch for these figures and prepare for changes.

B. *Rising or falling interest rates*
High interest rates make it more expensive to borrow money to open other offices, purchase technology or other capital equipment as well as to conduct an acquisition. Conversely, low interest rates offer a great opportunity to borrow money for capital expenditure and/or acquisitions.

C. *Inflation Rates*
High inflation rates usually create a threat to your agency due to the increased cost of doing business, conducting research, purchasing supplies, and paying wages and salaries of employees.

3. **Technological Forces** include scientific improvements and innovations that provide opportunities and/or threats for your agency. Recent technological innovations in computers, satellite networks, telemonitoring and other related areas have provided incredible opportunities for operational efficiencies, information storage, and actual client care.

4. **Social Forces** consist of the traditions, values, societal trends, and demographic trends of the culture and, in particular, the culture of your client base. Societal trends offer numerous opportunities and/or threats to your agency. For example the increasing number of people reaching sixty-five provides an incredible opportunity for your agency. Likewise, the trend toward single-family households also offers an outstanding opportunity for your agency. Other social forces that will affect your business include: an increase in life expectancy, shifts in the presence of women in the work force, the lack of and/or pressure on family-member care providers, and an overall increase in the culture for concern with — and a demand for — quality of life.

An Industry Analysis

Michael C. Porter of Harvard University, a leading authority on competitive strategy, contends that your agency's profit potential depends on five basic competitive forces within the Home Care Industry.

1. Threat of new competitors entering the marketplace
2. Intensity of rivalry among existing competitors
3. Pressure from substitute products or services
4. Bargaining power of the client
5. Bargaining power of the Home Care Agency

Let's look at each of these competitive forces.
(see diagram on page 23)

Threat of New Competitors Entering the Marketplace

The entry of a new competitor intensifies the fight for market share, resulting in overall lower market price and industry profitability. The two deterring factors that prevent or allow a company from entry into the marketplace are:

1. **The Level of Retaliation from the existing companies in the market.**
2. **Barriers to Entry**
   Naturally, barriers to entry are those factors that are likely to hold back new start-ups in your area — which may include your *own* business if you are just opening up or branching out. There are five major barriers to entry:

   Product Differentiation
   Strong brand identification of existing agencies forces a barrier — to overcome existing clients' loyalty.

FACTORS THAT AFFECT YOUR BUSINESS

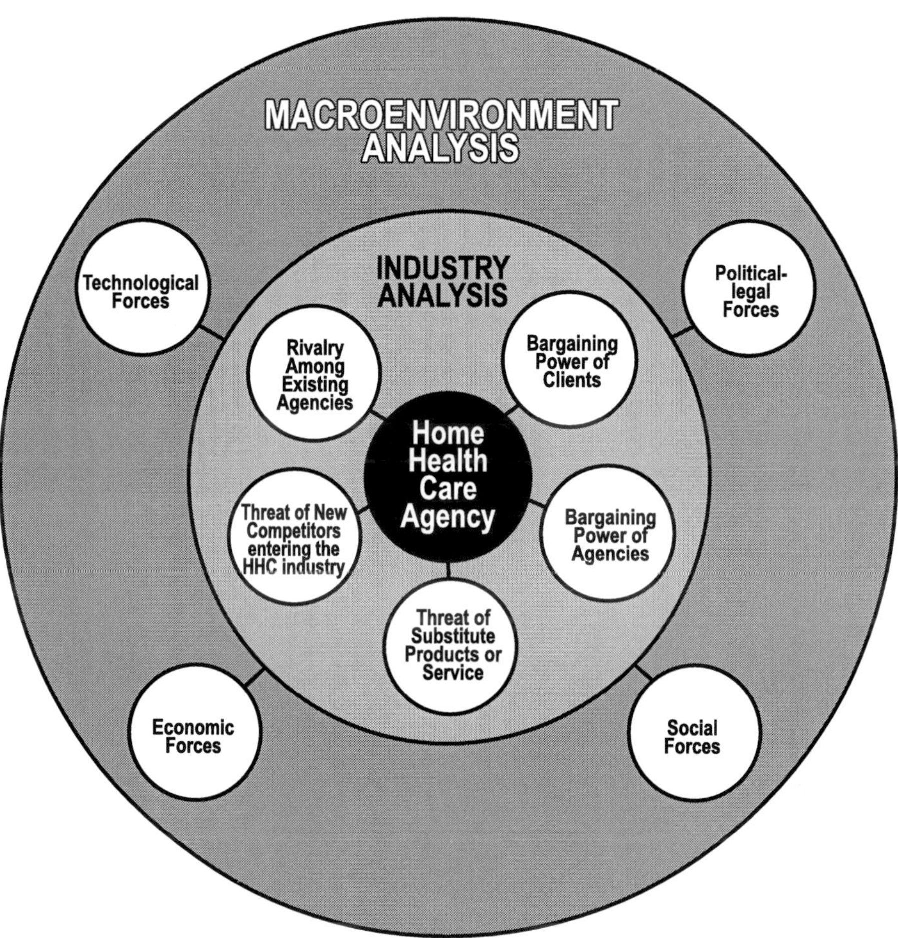

Brand identification and client loyalty are based on actual or perceived service differences, client services, or advertising.

Capital Requirements
The need to invest huge financial resources to enter the market creates a significant barrier to entry. Large amounts of capital are necessary for advertising, capital equipment, wages and salaries.

Switching Costs
Switching costs are the one-time costs that clients incur if they switch from receiving your services to receiving your competitor's services. If these switching costs are high, a new entrant must offer a major improvement in overall cost or performance to entice potential clients to change from their current agency.

Cost Disadvantage Independent of Size
Established agencies may have cost advantages that cannot be replicated by new entrants. These advantages may include proprietary product technology (such as scheduling software), a favorable location, and a head start on the "learning or experience curve" for that particular market area or niche.

Government Policy
Government can limit entry into the Home Care Industry with licensing requirements, such as the Certificate of Needs (C.O.N.).

Intensity of Rivalry among Existing Agencies

Competition among Home Care Agencies intensifies when one or more of the agencies identifies the opportunity to improve its position or feels competitive pressure from others. As a result of industry pressure, what often can follow are price cuttings, advertising battles, new service introductions, and increased client services. The intensity of competition is directly related to the following factors.

Number of Competitors

The number of agencies in a particular market and their sizes may determine the level of competitive rivalry. Markets with few agencies tend to be less competitive, but those that have a few large agencies are likely to be more competitive because each will strive to set the greatest market share.

Rate of Industry Growth

Agencies in markets that grow slowly are more likely to be highly competitive than agencies in rapidly growing markets. A booming market usually presents plenty of opportunity for many agencies to expand. However, in a slow-growing market, one agency's increase in market share comes at the expense of another agency's share.

Service Characteristics

When services can be differentiated from the competition, competition is less intense. Patients tend to have preferences and loyalties to a particular agency with differentiated services. But when services are less differentiated, a client's decision becomes based on price and service considerations, resulting in increased levels of competition.

Amount of Fixed Costs

Agencies with high fixed costs are under pressure to operate at nearcapacity levels to spread their overhead expenses over more areas of operations — which often leads to price-cutting and, in turn, greater competition in the market.

Height of Exit Barriers

Barriers to *exit* the Home Care Industry can be economic, strategic, or emotional factors, even if the agency is earning a small or negative return on its investment. Examples are labor agreements, strategic business relationships between inside divisions or other outside businesses, or the management's unwillingness to leave the Home Care Industry because of price, etc.

Diverse Competitors
Competitors often have diverse origins, strategies, and cultures, which usually result in different goals and ways of competing, and so they are more likely to cross paths and unknowingly challenge your position in the market.

Pressure from Substitute Products or Services

The Home Care Industry competes with firms in other industries that offer Substitute Products or Services — alternative products or services that satisfy similar client needs but are different in specific characteristics. Substitute services place a ceiling on the prices that Home Care agencies can charge. For example: Adult Day Care Centers offer a service for seniors that costs less than the price of Home Care, forcing Home Care agencies to keep their prices competitive.

Bargaining Power of the Client

Home Care clients affect the Home Care Industry through their ability to force down prices, demand higher quality or more services, and play agencies against each other. Home Care clients have the power to bargain:

- If the client has potential to supply their own nursing staff, i.e. hiring privately.
- If the Home Care market has many competing agencies and little differentiation.
- If changing agencies costs very little to the client.
- If the prices are outside the client's economic reach — providing an incentive to shop around for a lower price/ greater value, i.e. through hospitals, or assisted living.

Bargaining Power of the Home Care Agency

Agencies can affect their respective markets through their ability to raise prices or reduce the quality of service. Agencies can be powerful in the market:

- If there are few agencies in the particular marketplace.
- If the Agency's service is unique or can be differentiated from its competition and/or has built up a high cost for its clients to switch to another agency.
- If substitute services are not readily available.
- If the Agency's services are an integral part of the business of the Referral/Resource client, i.e. hospitals, nursing homes, etc.

It is quite evident from the Industry Analysis information that an agency could operate extremely profitably with:

- High entry barriers
- Low levels of competition in the marketplace
- Few or no substitute services
- Low bargaining power of clients
- Low bargaining power of other agencies
- High bargaining power for the Agency itself

On the other hand, an agency within a market with low entry barriers, high levels of competition, many substitute services, and high client and/or competition bargaining power would find it extremely difficult to be profitable.

To be successful, your agency/business must scan and research the Home Care Industry for opportunities and threats and internal strength and weaknesses. In short, your business must strategically position itself in the industry to be as profitable as possible.

Forecasting the Home Health Care Environment

Macro ("big picture") environmental and industry analysis is not as helpful to your agency if all it does is give you current trends. In order for this type of analysis to be an advantage to your agency, future trends and analyses must be identified or extrapolated through this process. The following are a few techniques (which you may come across in market studies, reports, economic articles, etc.) that your agency can use to help identify future trends and changes within the Home Care Industry: The Time Series Analysis, Multiple Scenarios, The Delphi Technique, and the Mind-Storming Technique.

Time Series Analysis

This analysis helps you to identify the effects of past and current market trends (such as life expectancy, changes in personal income, technological innovations, and number of competitors) on such variables as your agency's costs, sales, profitability, and market share over a specific period of time. This methodology also allows your agency to relate to such factors as seasonal fluctuations, weather conditions, and holidays to the firm's performance. Drawbacks: The basic problem with Time Series Analysis is that historical and current trends are based on a series of patterns made up of so many variables that a change in any *one* could significantly change the direction of the *trend*. Another potential weakness in a Time Series Analysis is that it provides quantitative data. Your agency should not place too much confidence in these results. The use of numbers for analysis can often not give a true picture of actual events/conditions in the market.

Multiple Scenarios

Due to the ever-changing macro environment and the industry itself, it is very difficult for your agency to formulate reliable assumptions, or predictions, based on most of the forecasting methods already discussed. One way to offset this challenge is to develop multiple scenarios about the future trends of the Home Health Care Industry.

I recommend that each member of the management team write several alternative predictions of the industry's future trends and events. For example, one scenario may present the most obvious and predictable future trends and events for the Home Care Industry. Another scenario may contain a more optimistic view — yet another a more pessimistic outlook. Look at all scenarios. Consider all, and then determine a plan of action for each case.

In developing scenarios, your management team must identify the key factors in the macro environment and industry that will affect your business. Identify any likely inter-relationships and predict their influence upon future trends (Industry regulations, technologies, political elections, etc.). These scenarios can help your agency develop possible contingency plans to prepare for the various market trends and events put forth in the scenarios.

Delphi Technique

For the Home Care Industry, the Delphi Technique is great to use in forecasting future trends and events. Choose several experts within the Home Care Industry and mail each of them a questionnaire asking for his or her opinions/estimates as to future trends and events that may affect the industry. (This does not need to be a "fancy" form — create your own, asking the questions informally and basing them on your particular market.)

Each respondent fills out the questionnaire without collaborating with any of the other experts and returns it to your agency. You then compile a *summary* of the respondents' answers and send it to each of them along with a second questionnaire. Some respondents may alter their opinions on the second questionnaire, after reviewing the opinions of the others.

Continue this process of responding – receiving – feedback – responding until a consensus has been reached. This can be an extremely valuable tool for your agency to predict future trends and to better position your agency in the marketplace.

Mind-Storming Techniques

Mind-storming is a non-quantitative technique that taps into people who are familiar with your industry and situation. These individuals are asked, as a group, to propose ideas — without judgment or critique. Set a time limit and a minimum number of ideas that everyone must come up with for the exercise. (I recommend fifteen to twenty minutes only. This forces everyone in the group to think fast and come up with as many ideas as possible.)

Once the initial time has expired, go through the list as a group and narrow down the ideas to half, based on the group's consensus. Continue this until you have at least twenty or so ideas that could be advantageous to your agency.

This technique is great to use with operating managers, directors, and nurses who tend to have more faith in "gut feelings" than quantitative analytical techniques.

The health care industry and the Home Care segments are changing so quickly that keeping up with trends and forecasting *future* trends will continue to be imperative.

Some things won't change, of course. People will always want attentive human contact, and people will always want to purchase services and products that improve their quality of life.

But you will not be able to deliver those services and products if you do not stay on top of market forces and trends, remain economically viable, and uniquely competitive.

CHAPTER SIX

Know Your Competition

Compete, don't envy.

— Moroccan proverb

Competitor Analysis

In order to determine your position within a given market area, it is important to investigate and analyze your competition. A Competitor Analysis should be conducted every six months by your agency. I have provided a Competitor Analysis format to assist you.

1. Choose five competitors within a forty-mile radius of your office or offices. In an urban or rural area you may choose to adjust the radius accordingly. The competitors you choose to analyze should be those Home Care companies with whom you continually compete for patients/clients. List their names at the top of the columns.

2. Determine the person(s) at your Home Care company who can best evaluate each competitor's operation. Determine how they will obtain the requested information. It may be advisable to obtain information on the phone prior to or after the visit.

3. Prepare for the evaluation by reviewing the information you currently have regarding a particular competitor. The following is a list of specific queries:
   - Geographical coverage
   - Hours of service (24 hours, 7 days a week, etc.)
   - Marketing strategy
   - Types of staff (RN, LPN, etc.)
   - Types of services offered
   - Specialty services offered
   - Rates for services
   - Number of nurses, homemakers, etc.
   - RN/patient ratios, LPN/patient ratios, Staff/patient ratios
4. When the form is completed, compare the information against your own company. How do they differ? What does your competitor have that your company does not?
5. Use the information you obtain to determine your strengths and weaknesses and to capitalize on the opportunities. Be sure to educate the sales team with your findings. If you identify weaknesses/barriers that may affect your ability to increase referrals, utilize the members of the Home Care team to focus on strategies to overcome the barriers.

COMPETITOR ANALYSIS WORKSHEET

Competitor Analysis		Your Agency	#1	#2	#3	#4	#5
Payor Mix	Private						
	Medicare						
	Medicaid						
	Other						
Geographical coverage							
Hours of Services (24 hours, 7 days a week etc.)							
Number of Nurses Homemakers, etc.							
RN, LPN, Staff/Patient Ratios							
Marketing Strategy							
RN Services							
	Rate						
LPN Services							
	Rate						
Attendent Services							
	Rate						
Homemakers							
	Rate						
Specialty Services							
	Rate						
Wound Care							
	Rate						
Private Duty Services							
	Rate						
Respite Care							
	Rate						
Assisted Care							
	Rate						
Live-In Companions							
	Rate						
Pediatric Services							
	Rate						
Special Geriatric							
	Alzheimer's Rate						
Home Infusion							
	Rate						
Respiratory							
	Rate						
HME							

75% OF ORIGINAL SIZE

CHAPTER SEVEN

Know (or Create!) Your Niche

Before you build a better mousetrap,
it helps to know if there are any mice out there.
— Mortimer B. Zuckerman

In order to know your most profitable position, or niche, in the market, you will need to analyze your company's strengths and weaknesses and how you differ from your competitors.

The point of analyzing your strengths and weaknesses is to enable your agency to take advantage of particular opportunities in the marketplace, to avoid or minimize external threats, and to position itself accurately in the market. Your agency's resources constitute its strength and weaknesses. They include human resources (experience, capabilities, knowledge, skills), organizational resources (the firm's systems and processes, including its strategies, structure, culture, purchasing, operations, financial base, research and development, marketing, information systems and central systems), and physical resources (geographical location, access to labor, technology, etc.). To have greater strength within your agency and to have a sustained level of performance and success in the marketplace, *all three resources* must be at optimal levels of performance.

S.W.O.T. Analysis

S.W.O.T. is an acronym for Strengths, Weaknesses, Opportunities and Threats. It is an assessment of the internal and external factors that can and do affect your agency. The *internal* capabilities of your Home Care Agency are analyzed by **strengths and weaknesses** and the *external* factors which impact your company are measured by **opportunities and threats.**

The S.W.O.T. analysis helps you pinpoint your resources and capabilities while pointing out your weak areas in order to minimize them. You must identify your potential opportunities based on your strengths and protect your Home Care Agency from competitor threats aimed at your weaknesses.

There are two forms to complete for the S.W.O.T. analysis. Form #1 lists several internal capabilities of your agency. Review each line item and place an X to define the item as a strength or weakness. You may want to ask other members of your team to assist you in analyzing your internal factors.

The second form lists external factors, which may be opportunities or threats to your company. (You may want to add additional items that may be unique to your community.)

Once you have completed the S.W.O.T. analysis, you will be able to begin formulating your goals and objectives for the upcoming year. As you progress in the planning process, you will also identify **strategies** necessary to assist you in accomplishing your goals and objectives.

SWOT ANALYSIS WORKSHEET

Strengths & Weaknesses

Location/Branch: ____________________

Strengths/Weaknesses (Internal)	S	W
Collateral Material (Marketing Material)		
Office Location - Condition, Cleanliness		
Marketing Program		
Referral Programs		
Diversified Services		
Quality of Nursing Care		
Competitive Pay Rates		
Experience of Staff		
Training Programs for Staff		
Staff Turnover		
Customer Service Orientation		
Name Recognition In The Market		
Recruitment Program		
Intake System, Back-Up Systems		
Sales Personnel		
Billing Systems		
Case Management		
Direct Insurance Billing		
Physicians - Quality/Support		
Referral Turnaround Time		
On-Site Evaluations		
Interdisciplinary Team Meetings		
24 Hour - 7 Days A Week - Nursing Services		
Medical Equipment Services		
Rehab Therapy Services		
Staff Moral		
Patient Satisfaction		
Employee Satisfaction		

* Once a weakness is identified, what actions are going to take place to overcome the weakness?

75% OF ORIGINAL SIZE

SWOT ANALYSIS WORKSHEET

Opportunities & Threats

Location/Branch (Continued): ____________________

Opportunities/Threats (External)	O	T
Location of Offices		
Perception of Care		
By Community / Clients		
By Referral Sources		
By Payors		
Relationship with Referral Sources		
Relationship with Referring Facilities		
Relationship with Physicians		
Relationship with Payors		
Competition - Other Home Care Companies		
Hospital based acute rehabilitation		
Assisted Living Facilities		
Payor		
Source of Referring Facilities		
Relationship with Case Managers		
Other Home Health Care Agencies		
Nursing Care Image		
Relationship with Local Community		
Medical Advisory Committee		
Government Regulations		
Labor Supply		
Demographic Trends		
Pricing / Billing Rates		

NOTE: In completing this form, decide what actions are necessary to minimize threats identified that could impact your business.

* What actions are necessary to minimize the threats identified at your agency?

75% OF ORIGINAL SIZE

Niche Marketing

Only giant companies have the resources necessary to market products or services to everybody. It is a mistake for small companies and entrepreneurs to market "one-stop-shopping." Although this may seem contrary to what has become "fashionable" in Home Care, you only have to look at the number of Home Care companies who have tried this marketing approach in the last five years to know that, without a great deal of capital, a company will fail if it attempts to market "broad."

Here are some criteria to consider:

- Size of the market
- Ability to reach the market affordably
- Ability to reach the market efficiently
- A known identified need
- Understanding of the market

"Specialization" or perceived specialization can turn an ordinary business into an extra-ordinary business, boost prices and margins, provide competitive differentiation and allow you to be a "big fish in a small pond."

Home Care Niche Markets can include:

- Pediatric Care
- Alzheimer's Care
- Rehabilitation
- Psychiatric Home Care
- Maternal and Child Health
- Custodial, Housekeeping
- Wound Care
- Services in Assisted Living Facilities

Determine the unmet needs in your community by meeting with the referral sources and asking them what Home Care services they are having difficulty finding for patients.

Determine the size of these "niche markets" and the potential contracts from these referral sources. Consider the barriers to entry into this market, i.e. specialized staff required and the availability of resources.

Determine your corporate expertise in this particular niche and develop a marketing strategy and projected budget.

Evaluate your potential return on investment.

If you identify more than one potential "niche" you wish to pursue, evaluate your strengths, weaknesses and your competitors' strengths in this particular niche, prior to investing time and money.

Proceed only when you have done your homework and are ready to lay groundwork.

Positioning a Small Home Care Company

There are many advantages of being a small Home Care provider. Home Care agencies are notably local-orientated businesses with distinct differences in each geographic location.

National companies — although they often advertise that each office is responsive to local needs — have built-in obstacles preventing them from being able to deliver quick response and implement programs specific to local needs.

Start with smallness and turn it into a *positive*. Make it work by stressing its advantages — *such as responsiveness and individual attention*.

Focus on your strengths, not your weaknesses. Your advertising should state: "*Our Home Care staff members are carefully screened and selected on the basis of their experience and their commitment to caring for people at home.*"

People want to do business with real people — not a corporation. Profile your owners, office staff and field staff in your ads and publicity. Put human faces in all your marketing campaigns.

Make the fact that you are *small* work as your *biggest* asset in niche marketing.

CHAPTER EIGHT

Determine Your Unique Selling Proposition (USP)

Always remember what you're good at and stick with it.

— Ermenegildo Zegna

A "Unique Selling Proposition," or USP, is a way of explaining your position against your competition. It's also a way of summarizing and communicating one of your major benefits. It should answer the question: "Why should I use your services versus your competitors ?"

Your USP should express the theme of your business, a product, or your positioning. Effective USPs are based on an exclusive niche, size, price, quality location, hours of operation, expertise, guarantee, customer service and so on.

As you concentrate on developing a new USP for your Home Care business, you can learn from examples of other companies. To hone your marketing mind, you must become

USP-sensitive and ask these questions about every business, product, and service you encounter in your daily activities:

1. Does this business have a USP?

2. If not, can I think of one for it?

3. If so, is there a way to improve it?

4. Are there any ideas here I can "steal" (incorporate) for my use?

Good sources for USP ideas are the Yellow Pages, newspapers or magazines. Get a large pile of blank 3"x 5" cards and start putting one fact, feature, benefit, promise, offer component, and idea on each card — until you have (over a series of brainstorming sessions) exhausted everything you know about your business and its competitors. Prioritize the items in order of their probable importance to your Home Care clients and their contribution to differentiating you from your competitors. Through this exercise, you can brainstorm on your own USP, plus create a supporting sales story and one or more related offers. Your USP should take advantage of an "opportunity gap" in your service area. Identify what your cleints, prospects and referral sources are not getting from your competitors and give it to them. Better yet, tell them with your USP. Think about it carefully. You should put your USP on all your marketing materials — even on your business card.

Remember, a USP should be limited to three sentences. The most effective are often only one sentence, but yours may well be three very short concise points. If your USP contains a promise such as a guarantee — *make sure you can deliver on your promise.*

Here are some examples of famous USPs:

- *Fresh Hot Pizza — delivered hot within 30 minutes, or it's free.* — Domino's Pizza

- *When it absolutely, positively has to be there overnight.* — Federal Express
- *The Ultimate Driving Machine.* — BMW
- *The Low Fare Airline* — Southwest

One-sentence Home Care Examples:

- *Quality Care in Your Own Home — Guaranteed!*
- *Professionals Caring for People at Home since 1965*
- *Providing Solutions for Your Home Care Needs 24 Hours a day, 7 days per week.*

CHAPTER NINE

Brand Your Business

Define yourself by what you do, by how you treat others, and how they see you.

— George F. Burns

In service marketing, almost nothing beats a successful brand. Name brands own about 90% of the market. In addition, national brands charge substantially more — up to 40% more than local or generic brands.

What is Branding?

Branding is the process of creating a singular idea or concept that you "own" inside the mind of your prospect. It is really as simple and as challenging as that.

Branding your Home Care agency should be the most important objective of its marketing strategy. All your marketing efforts really are about creating a brand in the mind of your prospects — thus, marketing is branding. These two concepts are so interconnected that it is impossible to separate them. Because everything that your agency does can contribute to its brand building process, marketing is an element that should not be considered independent from the rest.

Your agency, as I've already pointed out, should be in the business of marketing. *Marketing needs to be your agency's number one objective.* Why? Because marketing is responsible for building your brand in the mind of your prospects. Moreover, most services today are *bought* — not *sold* — thanks to the power of branding.

That old expression "Nothing happens until somebody sells something" has been replaced by today's expression:

> *"Nothing happens until somebody brands something."*

Branding "pre-sells" your service to the user by providing them with a feeling or an association that your service is the "best," the "cheapest," the "safest," etc., and greatly increases the chance of them buying your service. For example, Volvo has branded itself in the mind of its prospects to be the "safest" car on the road. Thus, if a prospect already has in his mind that Volvo is the safest car on the road and he wants to buy a safe car, then the chance of him being "pre-sold" to buy the Volvo over another car is much greater.

The same is true with the Home Care industry. If your agency can create a singular idea in the minds of its prospects, half your marketing work is done. For example, perhaps when your prospects see, hear or think of your agency they immediately think of a singular idea such as Senior Care, Shared Care, Pediatric Care, etc. By "owning" a word or singular idea in your prospect's mind, you will greatly increase your differentiation over competitors — and this will lead to a higher level of success.

What is a brand name?

A brand name is nothing more than a word or a symbol in the mind of your prospect. It is a warranty or a promise to your prospect that your service will live up to its name. Brands are especially important in the Home Care industry because very few agency services have warranties, and this leaves prospects only with "brands" on which to depend.

A very critical point in Home Care: *"A service is a promise, and building a brand builds your promise."*

The power of your brand lies in its ability to influence your prospects. A successful branding program is based on the idea of differentiation. It creates in the mind of your prospect the perception that there is no other service like your service.

Nearly every agency has a brand, an identity, a name, and a reputation. Brands provide functionality, images and experiences. Brands serve consumers by saving time, assuring a level of quality, and simplifying choice. The brand name — rather than the service — is now the primary reason your prospect will choose another agency over yours. The power of your brand proportionately relates to the amount of profits your agency will receive.

What's in a name?

The most important branding decision you will ever make is what to name your agency. In the long run, a brand is nothing more than a name. In the short-term, a brand needs a unique idea or concept to survive. It needs to be first in a new category. It needs to stick in your prospect's mind. Your brand is the essence of your agency. *Market share is not based on value, but on the power of the brand in the mind of your prospects.*

In the long run, a brand is not necessarily a higher-quality product, but a higher quality name.

One of the quickest ways to reach failure is to give your agency a generic name. For example: the generic name American Home Care is actually rather difficult to remember. It is too similar to U.S. Home Care, American Health Services, etc. I suggest that you avoid using a generic name for your agency. The problem with a generic name is its inability to differentiate the brand from the competition. In the home health industry you'll find agencies with generic names such as Tennessee Home Health, Tennessee Home Care Services, Home Care Services of Tennessee, Home Care Corporation of Tennessee, etc. I don't want to pick on any particular agencies, but will any of these generic brand names break into the mind of prospects and become a major brand? Probably not!

What I recommend that you do is find a regular word taken out of context and use it to connote the primary *benefit* of your brand. For example, "Partners Home Health" is a great name for a home health care agency because it is easy to remember and is catchy. "Partners Home Health" works as a successful brand name but "Tennessee Home Care Services" does not. Home Care agencies are recognized by prospects as being a "Partner" because of the nature of the business, so by taking the word "Partner" out of context and using it to connote the primary *benefit* of its brand, Partners Home Health was able to create a name that advertised a strong benefit, memorable — *and profitable.*

Think simple.

You want your name to be as short and as memorable as possible. Short names greatly improve word-of-mouth "marketing." However, don't use a monogram for your name.

People do not remember monograms. Monograms have no spirit, no attitude, no message, no promise, no warmth and no humanity — so give your service a name, not a monogram.

Think like a client and your brand will become successful. Your agency should limit its brand. That's the essence of branding. Your brand has to stand for something both simple and narrow in the mind of your prospect. The limitation is the essential part of the branding process. Limitation combined with consistency is what will build your brand.

Should you ever change your brand name?

I would only recommend *changing* your brand name if it is weak or nonexistent in the mind of your prospects. If you want to change your brand name, first look into the mind of your prospect. Where is your agency? Does your typical prospect bring you to mind when he thinks of Home Care? Perhaps your agency is not in the mind at all. If this is the case, then you can change your brand. But if you already have name recognition and some brand identity, then change your brand at your own risk. I highly recommend not changing.

Stand for something.

A well-known brand that doesn't stand for anything has no value. A brand that stands for something has value even if the brand is not well known. When your agency stands for something, it at least has the opportunity to create a powerful brand.

The most important aspect of your brand is its single-mindedness. For example — what is Ford? A large, small, cheap, expensive car or truck: This is an example of a burned-out brand that has lost its singularity. Loss of singularity can weaken your brand. If your agency currently provides home care services but is seeking to expand into other service categories such as home cleaning services, food catering services or any other service business that is not part of your primary attribute, *I recommend highly that you establish new brand names for these new services and keep them separate from your existing brand.*

When your agency can narrow its focus to just one service, i.e. senior care, it becomes a specialist rather than a generalist — and a specialist is perceived to "know more" and provide a higher quality service than a generalist. Don't confuse your prospects by being all things to all people. This can have a negative affect on your brand.

How do you create a brand?

Brands must be built, and this can be a time-consuming and expensive process. Today, brands are mostly built with publicity and maintained with advertising. Being first in a particular category can generate an enormous amount of publicity for your agency. Your local news media are more inclined to talk about what's new, what's first — not what's better. When your brand name can make news, it has a chance of generating publicity. What others say about your brand is much more powerful than what you can say about it yourself through advertising. That's why publicity can be much more powerful than advertising.

At first your brand may not mean anything to your prospects but over time your brand will come to represent a strong set of associations in your prospect's mind. A popular misperception that Home Care agencies have is that building a brand is simply a matter of developing some clever advertising to create a desired set of associations. Although advertising does play an important role in building your brand, your agency must have services, a price, and a delivery system that supports the image communicated through your advertising. The building of your brand should be directed by the vision of your agency's desired positioning in the marketplace, and must be implemented by all the decisions related to the marketing mix.

Essentially there are 3 types of branding:

- Functional Branding
- Image Branding
- Experimental Branding

Your agency has — or should have — an image brand. Image brands are often created in industries where services are relatively undifferentiated or quality is difficult to evaluate without prior usage, such as the Home Care industry. Image brands create value mainly by literally projecting an image to your target audience. Although image brands may be based on an extraordinary service, an image brand, such as yours, is distinguished from a competitor's because prospects "see it" as offering a unique set of associations — *or image.*

One of the most effective ways to create an image brand is through advertising. Your agency should advertise its services using images that appeal to the emotional needs of your prospects. For example: In your print and/or television advertising, I would recommend showing an image of an elderly person being assisted at home with her daily activities by one of your nurses. Make this a vivid shot of the elderly person relaxed and happy, perhaps along with the elderly person's son or daughter looking relieved because their parent is being well cared-for by your agency. This kind of image advertising creates an association in your prospect's mind that your agency can fill their emotional need. Before too long, your agency's name will project an image — and that image will cause people to think of your business when needing Home Care services. Image brands succeed when they make an emotional connection with the prospect.

Your brand can be represented visually as categories of thoughts or associations in your prospect's mind.

For example, consider "The Home Health Care Agency" (*see diagram below*). Through its line of services it has created a feeling of freedom, companionship, healthy living, happiness, etc. These thoughts are essential brand equity of "The Home Health Agency" and should be similar for your agency. For your brand to have value, these associations must become part of your prospect's mind. Does your Agency "Own" any of these words in the minds of your clients and prospects?"

DOES YOUR AGENCY "OWN" ANY OF THESE WORDS IN THE MINDS OF YOUR CLIENTS AND PROSPECTS?

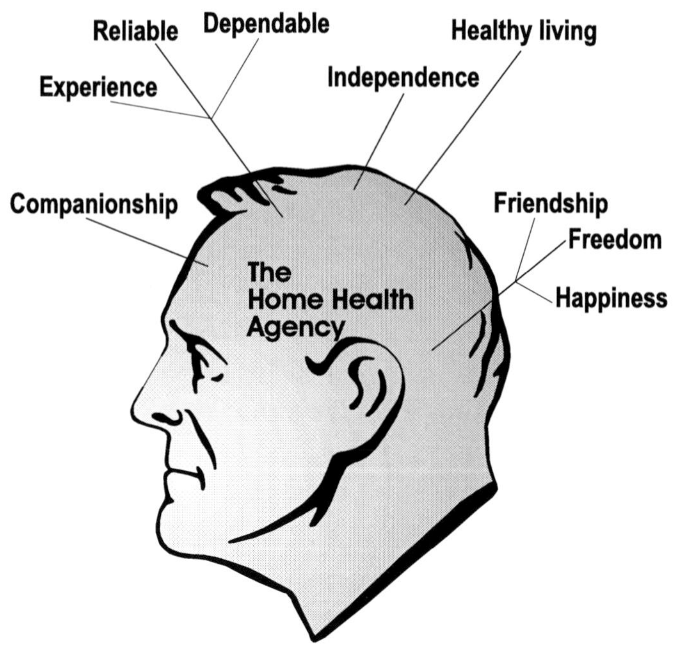

Be First.

The easiest way to get into your prospect's mind is to be first. The hard way to get into your prospect's mind is to be second. The reason that the first brand tends to maintain its leadership is because that name often becomes generic. Being second takes you nowhere. For example, the first person to fly across the Atlantic Ocean was Lindbergh. Who was second? That's my point. Nobody knows who second and third are. Develop your brand first because, in image branding, it is better to be first than it is to be better. It is much easier to get into your prospect's mind first than to try to convince them that you have a better service than your competitor who branded first.

What should your agency advertise if it is already #1? Brand leadership of course. Leadership is the single most important motivating factor in the mind of your prospect. For example, if your agency is the leading brand in Miami, Florida, you should say in your advertisements "Sunnyside Home Care Agency — *#1 in Miami Florida.*" Since most prospects want to have the best service, most prospects will want to use your brand because it is the leading brand.

There are also long-term benefits of being the leader. Once you get on top, it's hard to lose your spot. A widely publicized study of twenty-five leading brands in twenty-five different product and service categories in the year 1923 showed that twenty of the same twenty-five brands are still the leaders in their categories today. However, never assume that people know that your brand is the leader — you may need to remind them in your advertising. Note that most new prospects have no experience with Home Care and have little knowledge of available brands, so they will naturally gravitate to the leading brand — which is you.

If your agency can't be first in its particular category because another agency beat you to it, then I recommend that your agency create another category that you *can* be first in. For example, our agency had a situation where a larger competitor had a more popular brand in a particular market. All we did was develop another service category where we could be first. We marketed that we were the first agency to provide "Shared Care" in this particular market. Our agency quickly became the top brand in that market because we were first and had developed our brand.

When your agency introduces a new product, the first question that needs to be asked is not "How is our new service better or different from our competition?" but "What category is our new service *first* in?" Everyone is interested in what's new; few people are interested in what's better. When your agency is first in a new category, promote the category. If you are the first to introduce "Shared Care" in your market, then market "Shared Care."

Your agency will become incredibly successful if it can find a way to own a word in the minds of your prospects. Federal Express was able to put the word "overnight" into prospects' minds because it sacrificed its product line and focused on overnight delivery. Your agency can and should do the same. Your agency could "own" the phrases "senior care," "pediatric care" or "shared care" by focusing your marketing on one of these services. If your brand is second in the minds of your prospects then the marketing strategy of the leader must ultimately determine your agency's strategy — and this is not what you want. Your agency must discover the essence of the leader and present the prospect with an alternative — a new idea — a first in a field of services. Don't try necessarily to be better — try to be different, a leader.

CHAPTER TEN

Set — or Reset — Prices for Your Services

Standing in the middle of the road is very dangerous; you get knocked down by traffic from both sides.

— Margaret Thatcher

By far, the least fragile, least vulnerable, most desirable position to seek in your marketplace is being a "premium priced provider of premium service."

Do not assume that "logical" pricing is necessarily smart pricing. When selling Home Care services, there is a tendency to try to keep rates on the low end of the spectrum hoping this will increase market share.

Maybe your rates, which make you look like a good value, actually make you look second rate.

If no one ever complains about your rates, they may be too low. If almost everyone complains, they may be too high. Ten percent of potential clients and referral sources will complain about any price. Some people want a deal. Others are distrustful and assume every price is overstated.

Setting the Rates

If you are the higher-priced provider, most people *assume* you offer the best quality — a desirable position. Your marketing must stress that your rates are higher because you are providing them more value.

If you are the lower-priced provider, most people assume you deliver an acceptable product at the lowest cost — also an acceptable position. However, in the Home Care industry low prices may impede your ability to attract and retain the experienced staff you require.

If your prices are "in the middle" of the market, you are stating: "We are not the best, and neither is our price — both our service and price are pretty good." Not a compelling message. *If you are in the middle, you are competing with almost everyone.*

Specific Pricing Issues Affecting Home Care Companies

Cost shavers, particularly today in this tight labor market, find it harder to inspire employees as they see austerity as cheapness.

Do not hesitate to share with clients and employees that your prices include training, recruitment, insurances, supervisory and administrative salaries and overhead. Educate your clients as well as your referral sources.

Avoid charging for services by the hour whenever possible. Try to package services in units to avoid having competitors undercut by a few cents on the dollar.

Charge for knowing where to find the best employees — and retaining them. In Home Care "the companies that own the labor pool, own the market."

Pricing is part of Marketing.
A Home Care company's prices
must fairly reflect its value to the client,
or the service will fail.

CHAPTER ELEVEN

Have a Bold and Solid Guarantee

Golden rule principles are just as necessary in the operation of a business as scissors, twine and inventory.

— J.C. Penney

"Our staff are carefully selected, screened and supervised. If you are not 100 percent guaranteed with our services, we want to know and we will refund your costs and find a replacement within 24 hours."

How many Home Care companies that you know of offer this type of guarantee?

Offering guarantees has not been a practice in the Home Care industry. However, this is changing as more and more people begin to pay for in-home services out of their own pocket. Consumers are demanding guarantees.

If your company's name is not well known, this is one way to make a very bold statement. It does, however, carry the responsibility of living up to a commitment. *Don't advertise a guarantee unless you are 100 percent committed to honoring it.*

Most, if not all, Home Care companies would absolutely refund a client's money if a client were unhappy and complained about the service. Why not tell a client or referral source right up front that this is your practice? — or better still, put it in writing!

Why is a guarantee so important?

If your agency advertises a "satisfaction-or-your-money-back-with-a-smile" guarantee, imagine the confidence it will create with prospects and clients. Providing your service is what you do best — so why not guarantee it? Even if someone *does* have a complaint, they most likely will end up as one of your best ambassadors:

> "You know The Home Care Agency? Well, I wasn't happy with the new homemaker that was caring for my mother and I told them about it. They immediately sent another homemaker out to the house for me to meet. This quality of service is tops and they aim to please. It must have been an isolated incident. I would recommend them to look after anyone's loved one."

This is much better than having a dissatisfied client say "I'll never use The Home Care Company again." What's more, dissatisfied clients tell, on average, 20 other people of their bad experience. Can you afford this? Absolutely not — especially if you operate in a small community.

Effect on Employees

You will be amazed how having a guarantee will affect employees. When you inform all your employees that the company's policy is to "guarantee" that all clients will be satisfied or their money will be refunded, it sends a very powerful message of just how committed you are to ensuring client satisfaction.

Think about it in this way: Would you get your carpets cleaned without a guarantee? Why should anyone accept anything less from a Home Care provider?

You may think that by providing a guarantee many people will take advantage of you. But in reality very few people will and for the few that do — it will be offset by the overwhelming increase in business that you will receive by removing the *risk* from your prospects and putting it onto you. This single strategy will differentiate you from your competition and increase your market share virtually overnight.

CHAPTER TWELVE

Start Collecting Testimonials

The eyes believe themselves,
the ears believe other people.

— Ella Wheeler Wilcox

What *others* say about your company is infinitely more believable than what *you* say about your company.

Many clients and families like to take the opportunity to write and thank you for providing services and to compliment your staff. These "testimonials" can be a very powerful marketing tool and most companies underestimate just how valuable they can be.

Consider:

- Testimonials are one of the first things a person reads in an ad or brochure.
- Testimonials add credibility.
- You can never use too many testimonials.

Start Gathering — Now!

You can solicit testimonials by providing clients, families and referral sources with a questionnaire. Ask for permission to use their testimonials in your advertisements and marketing material. You can ensure them you will use their initials and will not disclose names or other personal information.

Talk to your clients — those who you know really love your staff and your company. Don't ask them to write a testimonial, per se. Give them a preprinted form to fill out. This will make it much easier for your client to complete and you will get the information you need. Include a form in your "New Client Kits" (covered in a Part III) and make sure your staff knows that you want these returned to the office.

- Read every testimonial form that comes back.
- Make sure all your staff read them.
- Start a three-ring notebook of your testimonials and keep it updated.

Put copies of the very best testimonials in your newsletters, post them on your web site and include them in your brochures. *They will greatly enhance your marketing materials — and increase your response rate.*

What Testimonials Should Say

- Have at least one testimonial for each benefit of your service.
- The testimonial should be used to create credibility.
- Include the quoted person's full name. This will add credibility.
- If appropriate, include the service they received, i.e. homemaking, shared care, pediatric care.

CHAPTER THIRTEEN

Look Around, Take Notes

Ideas are the currency of the 21st Century.

— Brian Tracy

Model the Marketing Ideas of Others

Modeling ideas from others can be very profitable for your agency. I'm not talking about stealing or plagiarizing your competition's successful marketing campaigns. *What I mean is that it is extremely valuable to learn from others.* Take their good ideas and adapt them to fit your agency's marketing objectives or strategies.

This doesn't necessarily mean modeling from other Home Care agencies, although it is a good idea to take notes on how other agencies position themselves — especially when you attend local health fairs, trade shows, etc. Use and adapt marketing ideas that are working for others whether they come from the Home Care industry or the carpet cleaning industry. If the idea is profitable in one service sector it may well be profitable in another. This is the "law of success." Model the actions of one and reap the same rewards. It's that easy!

A great example of this was in the fast food industry. Do you think McDonald's invented the drive-thru-window? No! The banking industry was the first to introduce this convenient service. An executive of McDonald's merely identified this idea as an opportunity, and the rest is marketing history. It changed the face — *and the pace!* — of the fast food industry.

You can get great marketing ideas from just about anywhere. Always be looking out for successful marketing ideas that you can apply to your agency. Read the direct mail offers that you receive in the mail. Look to see what new techniques the large national direct mail companies are using. Remember, they have large budgets and have probably tested their mailings, so the chances are high that some of these strategies will work for your agency.

Attend the meetings and functions of the associations you belong to. You might get a lot of new and exciting marketing methods to try from other Home Care agencies that you meet at these functions.

A Note to consider: Some Home Care agencies won't be willing to share any of their profit-producing marketing ideas with you if they are competing in the same market. But some will — and these are the ones that you want to form relationships with.

Why reinvent the wheel when it has already been created? Save your agency time, money and the grief of using unproven marketing strategies by adapting proven techniques — from this manual or other businesses — that might be profitable for your agency. Be humble and keep your eyes open. Your agency will be successful...faster!

CHAPTER FOURTEEN

Develop Your Marketing Plan

The great thing in this world is not so much where we are, but in what direction we are moving.

— Oliver Wendell Holmes

It is critical that you develop a marketing plan for your business in order to have a blueprint to follow and to enable you to evaluate and monitor what is working for your business.

The purpose of your initial brainstorming will be to flesh out the variables that will directly affect to whom you will market, where you'll market, and how you'll market. Brainstorm, brainstorm, and then brainstorm some more. You may end up writing similar paragraphs and ideas for pages and pages. That's OK. The point is to get at the core of who you are, what purpose can you serve that greatly benefits others, and where you want to be. Marketing is your vehicle for getting there.

You will find a series of worksheets in the last chapter, "Putting Pen to Paper," which you can use to refine your brainstorming notes. These worksheets will help stimulate your creative thinking and generate new ideas.

Develop client profiles.

Draw up profiles of what you envision to be your typical clients. For example, many Home Care clients are elderly females who live alone and have more than one physical ailment. Remember also that your target audience must include the children of prospective clients who are typically forty-five to sixty years old. Include MD's and other referral sources on your list.

Clarify the benefits you offer.

When you have clearly focused on your market, you can clarify your market position. Then you should measure the position against four criteria:

1. Do our services offer a benefit that our target audience really wants?
2. Are they honest-to-goodness benefits?
3. Do our services/benefits truly separate us from our competitors?
4. Are they unique and/or difficult to copy?

Make a list of at least twenty-five features that describe your business. Do not edit. Write down everything you can think of. Then, next to each feature, write down how this feature is a benefit to your clients.

Define your Image and Brand.

What is so special about your business? What do you offer that your competitors do not? (What is your USP — Unique Selling Proposition?) What are your clients' unique needs?

It is possible to build an entire marketing plan based on one difference between you and your competitors. (Examples: Hours of service, staff selection, insured and bonded staff and services, fluent in languages other than English, special training, etc.) Whether it is a specialty service, convenience of hours or service, or some other unique feature, take advantage of this difference.

Develop a focus group of your colleagues, employees and former or present clients to help validate your information and to gain valuable feedback.

Define your Purpose.

Your key message must convey to the prospective client that you have the solution to their problem. Here are some creative ideas that might help to describe the purpose of your business:

- We provide solutions to enable people to remain in their own homes when they are convalescing.
- We provide clinical staff to assist in a patient's rehabilitation and recovery.
- We offer alternatives to institutional long-term care.
- We specialize in care and assistance for children with special needs.
- We have committed, caring staff available to assist seniors with daily living.

You must develop a message that conveys what makes your company special and what makes your employees special.

Your Positioning Statement

Your finished marketing plan, which lays out your yearly advertising plan, may well run ten pages. At first though, try to state it in one paragraph. This initial "mini-marketing plan" will become your "first draft" positioning statement. Study the marketing options presented in Parts II and III of this manual, and then take another look at your positioning statement before you write out your final yearly plan.

Create your positioning statement with seven sentences:

1. Explain the purpose of the strategy.
2. Explain how you'll achieve this purpose — through your competitive advantage and benefits.
3. Describe your target market or markets.
4. List the marketing weapons you think you'll employ. (This will be your longest sentence.)
5. Describe your niche.
6. Describe your identity — and brand image — of your business.
7. State your marketing budget, expressed as a percentage of your projected gross revenues. (When planning your marketing budget, figure on spending two to five percent of gross sales.)

An example of a positioning statement for a marketing plan:

> The purpose of Our Home Care Company is to provide professional home care services tailored to the individual health needs of our clients. This will be accomplished by positioning Our Home Care Company services as being valuable to clients and referral sources. The target market

will be those who require home care services or who have a family member who requires home care services.

The marketing tools we plan to use include classified advertising in magazines, newspapers and on-line communication, direct mail, promotion to referral sources, participating in health fairs and seminars, and setting up a web site linked to other health care information sources. The niche that Our Home Care Company occupies is a service sector that responds to a patient's needs with empathy. Our identity and brand image will be one of compassionate expertise, flexibility and quick response to client requests. Our marketing budget will represent 5% of our revenue.

Get feedback.

Once you have completed writing your marketing plan (it may not be the final draft), and certainly before you roll out a new service, do some informal "testing." Get feedback from former and existing clients, referral sources and staff.

Give your marketing plan to everyone in your company as well as close business associates to review. This will help your staff get a better understanding of your focus. It will also help to solicit a number of new ideas based on their perspective of working in your business.

Provide employees with an opportunity to offer suggestions and ideas on the marketing plan — how to improve service delivery, reach prospective clients and referral sources, etc. Ask for their help. You may even want to develop a questionnaire asking for their feedback and ideas. Offer employees an incentive to complete the questionnaire or a prize for the best suggestion used. Make sure you recognize employees who give input. If you have a newsletter (covered in a later chapter) note their contributions here. Send thank you letters to all employees who complete the questionnaire telling them how much you value their input.

Provide an orientation for all employees regarding your marketing and promotional program. You must get employees to support your efforts and become enthusiastic.

Once the foundation is set, begin building.

Read the Manual!

Part II of this manual deals directly with advertising materials and media placed marketing. Part III deals with indirect marketing and public relations marketing — equally necessary for maximum success. To fully lay out your yearly plan, you will need to read through the entire manual to know all your options and to generate some great ideas. However, here are some brief pointers as you are developing initial drafts.

When deciding which of your marketing ideas to launch first, pick the one or two that you believe will be most likely to succeed. This will make you more confident about tackling the other items on your list. If you are just starting out in business, focus on one specific market segment. (You *can* try marketing ideas that have worked well for other Home Care companies. However, they should be tailored to your specific needs.)

If you feel that private duty companion or attendant care services are needed in your area, then focus on where your potential clients live and identify the referral sources that could use your services — such as physicians, clinics, senior centers, churches, trust officers, etc.

- First impressions count! When it comes to brochures and business cards, keep this in mind at all times.
- Promotional materials should stress your uniqueness. Copy should appeal to a potential client's unique needs.
- Testimonials in your marketing materials must demonstrate exactly how your services helped the client.

Give promotional copy a sense of urgency. Direct your advertising and marketing materials as if you're speaking to one person at a time. Make the reader feel special. Writing copy in *second person* is very effective (i.e., "You will…", "Your loved ones…" or "Take a moment to improve the quality of your life. Call today…"

Proofread every piece of written material that you send out. Never allow anyone to mail out promotional material before it has been proofed several times.

You must also convey in your message that you really understand clients' needs — that you have a qualified experienced staff that will provide individualized attention.

Let potential clients know about your specific qualifications, years in business, insurance coverage, screening, and supervision of employees.

Offer a commitment or guarantee and stand behind this. Many HomeCare companies hesitate to offer a written guarantee because they fear it willcost them money if a client complains and doesn't want to pay for a homemaker who didn't perform the assigned duties or meet their expectations. Remember, if the client is dissatisfied, they will tell at least eighty people directly or indirectly that your company did not live up to their expectations.

CHAPTER FIFTEEN

Stay On Track

Victory belongs to the most persevering

— Napoleon Bonaparte

Commit to working on your business.

Marketing does not end once the plan is set. It is a year-long process of tracking, review, and reassessment. And no one else will do it if you don't.

Every day, set aside a block of time to devote to reviewing your marketing. Make sure that you also plan in advance for special events and promotions. Plan at least a month ahead of a big promotion before introducing new services.

It is imperative that you remain consistent in the execution of your marketing and promotion.

Stick to your plan. Don't stop doing what you have laid out in your plan. Consistency and commitment are the keys to success.

Give your marketing plan at least 60–90 days to show results, and review your marketing plan at least once every month.

Check your progress against your marketing efforts of the last month. For the first three months, focus all your marketing on one specific group or service. Track your results for the following 90 days to see how this marketing decision increases your business.

It becomes very tempting to just "copy" your competitors and to change direction once you get started. Don't become discouraged when you don't see results overnight. Stick to your plan and wait at least 90 days to re-evaluate your direction.

Remember — it will take time for the marketplace to respond to your advertisements and promotions. By remaining consistent, you will eventually begin to see your time and investment pay off.

Many times after we initiated a promotional ad campaign to introduce a new service or after opening a new office, we would be disappointed when the phone wouldn't ring off the hook right away. Keep your enthusiasm level up. It takes time and when the phone does start ringing, be prepared! It was our experience that referrals would come in waves — usually on a Friday before a long weekend when your staff is ready for vacation!

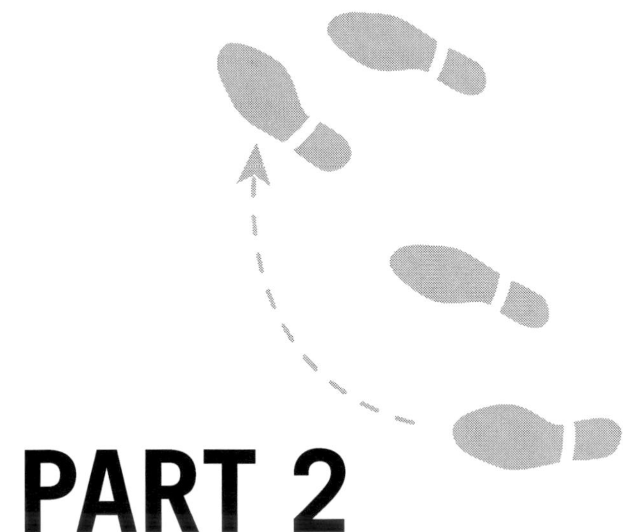

PART 2

Establishing Your Advertising Plan and Your Presence in the Market

CHAPTER SIXTEEN

Plan Your Yearly Advertising

Define your business goals clearly so that others can see them as you do.

— George F. Burns

You've put together the groundwork for your marketing plan. You're ready to plan your advertising. Now ask yourself: *What is the purpose of advertising?* To get new clients? Yes, partly.

The purpose of advertising *is* to get new clients, but you also need to get referrals from these new clients and then get referrals from the referrals. This is how your company will build up the "critical mass" (number of clients to provide you with enough referrals to sustain your business) it needs to make new profits. *However*, the only way that your company is going to *get* new clients is through advertising.

Budget for marketing.

I recommend that *every year* your company put together a specific goaloriented marketing plan for the entire year that fits within your current marketing budget. If you don't have a marketing budget — *get one!*

When planning your marketing budget, figure on spending two to five percent of gross sales. (This will depend on your margins and available cash flow.)

Try to figure out how much the competitors in your market area are spending. Make sure you are allotting at least as much as they are spending.

Why budget? Because advertising is crucial. You must advertise your company if you are going to bring in new business and keep referrals coming in, or sooner or later you won't have any new business or referrals!

Advertising is the primary vehicle for your business to communicate its services to the private-pay market. It is a form of mass communication that allows your business to clone its sales presentation and deliver it to a large number of targeted prospects all at once. Nothing else communicates your services, your value, and your image to your target audience like well-planned, well-placed advertising. *Advertising both informs and transforms your service by creating a message that goes beyond straightforward facts.*

Direct and Indirect Action Advertising

Advertising "gets things moving!" — either directly, or indirectly.

Direct action advertising — or direct response advertising — can produce an immediate response from your target audience. For example: If you mail out a direct mail piece that contains a coupon for a 50% discount on a first visit with a sales expiry date of 15 days or so, you should expect an immediate response from some of your target audience.

Indirect action advertising is designed to create demand for your services over a long period of time. For example: if you write a weekly column for the newspaper that consistently provides the local community with interesting, informative health care information, you are also branding and positioning your company as an expert in this field. Then, when your readers need Home Care services some day, they are most likely to call *your* company — the one they already know.

What other vehicle could provide you with these benefits?

Advertise, advertise and keep advertising. It's the fuel for your company's growth.

Diversify Your Marketing

There are many ways to market and advertise your services. Should you pick just one? Several? I recommend that you use a multi-tiered approach to your marketing strategies. Establish your identity pieces (business cards, brochures) and target which media best serve your budget, your goals, your message and your particular market. Diversification increases new business and referrals — and it also allows you to test and track several advertising avenues.

Ideally, you should consider all venues and media to market your business:

1. Direct Mail pieces — brochures, flyers
2. Signage and Billboards
3. Print — newspapers, magazines, newsletters, trade journals
4. Local Radio — advertisements and talk shows
5. Local Television — advertisements and talk shows
6. Web Site and Internet Banner Ads
7. Existing Clients and Referral Marketing
8. Tradeshows — local, regional, national
9. Network marketing through organizations, clubs
10. Public Relations — hosting or sponsoring local social events

Why do you need to diversify your marketing?

As the old adage goes — "don't put all your eggs into one basket." And just like your stock portfolio adviser says: *Diversify, diversify, and diversify!* Diversification will reduce your level of risk and provide a steady influx of new business from different sources. Sales is the key to the success of your business, so you must have multiple strategies working at all times to provide your company with maximum sales.

Sometimes one strategy might take longer than anticipated to generate your forecasted sales. If you have a couple other strategies in place, staggered to hit different market segments, you will have a more consistent level of sales, and you'll reduce your risk of huge dips that could have a major impact on cash flow.

How do I diversify my marketing strategies?

At the beginning of the year sit down with your marketing managers/team and plan out your marketing strategies for the year. I recommend that you use plenty of notebook paper plus the worksheets provided in chapter 48: "Putting Pen to Paper."

Key: You must plan your marketing strategies at the beginning of the year. This will help you establish a budget, with clear objectives and goals written down. Then, everyone in the organization will have a road map of what needs to be done and where the company is going. Just by writing down your goals, you will have an eighty percent chance of success!

Finding one particular strategy that works great for you doesn't mean that you should terminate your other strategies. Stick to your original marketing strategies that you set at the beginning of the year and you will experience greater results than you would have ever imagined.

The biggest problem that most agencies face is failure to stick to their original plan and starting a "shotgun" or panic strategy when sales are down — dumping a huge amount of money into one strategy and waiting for the calls. When a company is already suffering from a cash-flow problem from lack of sales, this panic strategy is an expensive way to yield very few results. Remember, it can take 30 days or more for a new strategy to take hold.

A diversified strategy can target several market segments at once — whereas the shotgun strategy targets a single segment. A diversified strategy also provides you with the benefit of having your audience experience repetition of your marketing, which is by far the most effective strategy to get the market to recall and identify your company name.

CHAPTER SEVENTEEN

Track Your Results

The toughest thing about being a success is that you've got to keep on being a success.

— Irving Berlin

Why do you need to track your marketing results?

If you don't know what's working and what's not, you will have no way to focus your marketing efforts and will lose *significant* potential business down the road.

You can't guess whether something is working or not. You must keep track of the numbers and let them tell you what is more successful.

Let me give you an example.

Campaign I: A local newspaper ad.

- It costs $2,000 to run it in the Sunday paper.
- Circulation of the paper is 15,000.
- You get 20 new clients from the ad

Campaign II: A direct mail piece to referral sources.

- It costs $6,132 to send to 1,000 prospects.
- You get 15 new clients from the mailing.

What campaign gave you the most revenue? At first it may appear that Campaign I gave you the most revenue — but look at the rest of the numbers.

Campaign I: Each of the 20 new clients generated an average of 10 hours/week

- 10 hours x $30/hr (nursing per hour rate) = $300/week per client
- 3 clients will have services for 12 months and 17 will need 8 weeks.
- 3 clients at $300/week x 52 weeks = $46,000
- 17 clients at $300/week x 8 weeks = $40,800

Your total gross revenue from Campaign I: $86,800

Campaign II: Each of the 15 new clients generated an average of 15 hours/week

- 15 hours x $30/hr (nursing per hour rate) = $450/week per client
- 8 will have services for 12 months, 3 for 6 months, 4 for 2 months.
- 8 clients at $450/week x 52 weeks = $187,200
- 3 clients at $450/week x 26 weeks = $35,000
- 4 clients @ $450/week) x 8 weeks = $14,400

Your total gross revenue from Campaign II: $236,600

Let's look at the results:

Campaign II pulled the greatest revenue with $236,600. Campaign I pulled less with $86,800. Even after removing the initial up-front costs for the marketing campaigns, Campaign II still generated the most profit.

This example shows you *why* you must keep close track of your numbers. Sometimes it may look as if one campaign is pulling better than another until you start to track the results. You should track the results of *all* your marketing efforts to determine if you should continue to use the same campaign or if you need to make some changes to pull a better return.

Sometimes even the best marketing ideas — with the best intentions, best efforts, outstanding services, apparent market, and many other positive factors — will not produce positive returns. At some point in time, you have to stop pouring good money in after bad results and go onto your next marketing campaign.

Tracking your marketing results can be reduced to one simple formula:

How many dollars did your company spend, and how many dollars did your company make from that marketing outlay?

Marketing Tracking Sheet

The purpose of the "Marketing Tracking Sheet" (see example provided at the end of this chapter) is to help your company determine the results from each of your marketing campaigns. The results from this sheet will help you:

- Determine your return on investment for each particular marketing project.

- Determine the true cost of each project.
- Decide whether to continue to use the campaign or move on to another one.

Calculating the Project Cost

The Marketing Tracking Sheet includes a section to record the Project Costs for the promotional campaign. It is important to calculate the cost to acquire your new client. This helps in determining the net profit your agency will make from each new client.

Project Cost — Production and mailing of 10,000 Brochures

1. Project Design and Printing $2,732
2. Postage (1st class) $0.34 x 10,000 = Mailing Cost $3,400
3. Total Costs $6,132
4. Cost per 1000 = $613.20, Cost per unit = $0.6132

Logging Results & the Average Lifetime Net Value of a Client

To log your results:

- Put the number of new clients you generate in the "new clients" box.
- Put in the projected average Lifetime Net Value of the client in the money column.
- Under each entry you will put in the cumulative amount for both "New Clients" and "$" up to that date.

In order to log the projected value of each client, you need to figure out what the average client lifetime value is for your agency. For the purpose of this exercise let's use the following as the average lifetime value of client:

1. New clients use *6 hours per week of services @ $30/hr = $180/week
2. $180/week x **52 weeks = $9,360 for the year
3. Thus, on average, each new client that your agency receives is worth approximately $9,360 to you.

   *(Assuming rates for skilled homemaking services)

   **(Assuming 52 weeks is the average length of service for your clients)

Once you have figured out what the average new client is worth, you can take this figure $9,360 and subtract your overhead costs. For this exercise we will assume overhead runs 85% of gross — or $7,956 — plus the cost of advertising to retain this new client — which is $6,132 divided by 10,000 = $0.61.

$7,956 + $0.61 = $7,956.61 (Total Outlay)

Now take the total lifetime value of your new client at $9,360 and subtract your total outlay of $7,956.61 You get $1,403.39 as the Lifetime Net Value of a client for this campaign.

This how much you will net on average for each new client, and it goes into the money column. Thus if you get *two* new clients on Day One, put $2,806.78 (which is $1,403.39 x 2) into the money column. Be sure to input the cumulative totals under each day in the money column to give you daily totals. Also do the same for the number of new clients.

Now our calculations have shown us that the two orders you received on Day One are worth $1,403.39 each, or a grand total of $2,806.78 to start paying you back the $6,132 in advertising you just laid out. So input the total $2,806.79

next to the two orders in the money column, and wait to see what the next day brings you.

At the end of the month you will have a total for both the number of new clients that your agency received and total money/sales for that particular marketing tool.

This method is great for providing your agency with a clean and quantitative look at how successful your marketing efforts really are. It also gives you the opportunity to compare one marketing campaign/tool against another or the same marketing campaign run at different times.

Always record each day's data that same day. For example, if you receive a phone call from a new client in the morning wanting to use your services and you receive another call in the afternoon from a new client also wanting to retain your services, you must record both on that same date. Do not record one entry for that day and the other for the next day. This will confuse you if you refer back to compare against the same publication or mailing when you're running the same publication or list again. In order to have accurate data to both quantity/track and to compare results, you must be consistent with your data entry. By being consistent you will have more accurate comparisons, and will make better marketing decisions.

This system only requires a few minutes each day to input data for any one advertisement, any one mailing, etc. A clerical employee can easily handle the daily data input. However, I strongly recommend that you review the "Marketing Tracking Sheet" personally every single day. You should have complete and immediate control of the marketing results yourself.

Advertising becomes income — and if it's successful, profits too. And you want to closely see the evolution of those profits daily.

Calculate Return on Your Brochure Expenditure

It is essential to calculate your "break-even" point in order to know if your marketing campaign is successful or not. The following example, using the example promotional campaign figures, calculates what your break-even point is:

$6,132 (campaign costs) divided by $1403.39 (Lifetime Net Value) = 4.36. Therefore, 4.36 new clients are required to break even on the campaign.

- To realize 50% profit: 4.36 x 1.5 (4.36 + 50%) = 6.55 new clients required.
- To realize 100% profit: 4.36 x 2 (4.36 + 100%) = 8.72 new clients required.

Calculate Return on Ads

The same calculations work as well for an ad as they do for direct mail. Let's say the ad cost was $2,000 and your services yield $1,403.39 net profit per new client on average. All you do is divide the ad cost of $2,000 by the $1,403.39 net profit per new client and this comes out to 1.42 new clients needed to break even on the ad. If you want to figure out a 50% return, just multiple 1.42 by 1.5 to get 2.1 new clients. For a 100% return, just double the 1.42 to get 2.8 new clients needed.

MARKETING TRACKING SHEET

Marketing Tool: ______________ Headline: ______________

Publication/Newspaper: ______________ Issue: ______________ Size: ______________

Mailing List: ______________ Mailing Date: ______________ Quantity: ______________

Notes:	Project Costs		Analysis	
	Project Design Cost	$ ______	Cost per 1000	______
	Ad Cost (Placement)	$ ______	Cost per Unit	______
	Printing	$ ______	Break even	______
	Mail Fulfillment Cost	$ ______	50% return	______
	Postage	$ ______	100% return	______
	TOTAL	**$ ______**		

	Jan.		Feb.		Mar.		Apr.		May		June		July		Aug.		Sept.		Oct.		Nov.		Dec.	
Date	# New Clients	$	# New Clients	$	# New Clients	$	# New Clients	$	# New Clients	$	# New Clients	$	# New Clients	$	# New Clients	$	# New Clients	$	# New Clients	$	# New Clients	$	# New Clients	$
	cumulative	cumulative	cumulative	cumulative	cumulative	cumulative	cumulative	cumulative	cumulative	cumulative	cumulative	cumulative	cumulative	cumulative	cumulative	cumulative	cumulative	cumulative	cumulative	cumulative	cumulative	cumulative	cumulative	cumulative
1																								
2																								
3																								
4																								
5																								
6																								
7																								
8																								
9																								
10																								
11																								
12																								
13																								
14																								

75% OF ORIGINAL SIZE

MARKETING TRACKING SHEET—SIDE#2

	Jan.		Feb.		Mar.		Apr.		May		June		July		Aug.		Sept.		Oct.		Nov.		Dec.	
Date	# New Clients	$	# New Clients	$	# New Clients	$	# New Clients	$	# New Clients	$	# New Clients	$	# New Clients	$	# New Clients	$	# New Clients	$	# New Clients	$	# New Clients	$	# New Clients	$
	cumulative	cumulative	cumulative	cumulative	cumulative	cumulative	cumulative	cumulative	cumulative	cumulative	cumulative	cumulative	cumulative	cumulative	cumulative	cumulative	cumulative	cumulative	cumulative	cumulative	cumulative	cumulative	cumulative	cumulative
15																								
16																								
17																								
18																								
19																								
20																								
21																								
22																								
23																								
24																								
25																								
26																								
27																								
28																								
29																								
30																								
31																								

75% OF ORIGINAL SIZE

CHAPTER EIGHTEEN

Business Cards

First impressions count!

The business card is of the most overlooked marketing tools by Home Care agencies. This will probably be the most important printed marketing tool that your agency will create. *Make your business card pay its own way!* Most business cards don't serve as marketing tools because they don't say anything to your prospective clients — they don't do anything to make clients call you.

Your business card should tell why your agency is different and better from your competition, and give your prospects a reason to call your agency.

Why is your Business Card the best promotional device?

- Often the first (sometimes the only) promotional material that your company produces.
- Often the first (sometimes the only) promotional material that your prospective clients will see.

- Inexpensive advertisement — a box of cards can go a long way!
- Projects an image of your agency — if you have a well designed card it will portray the image of your agency.
- Easy-to-use sales tool — uncomplicated, flexible, easy to pass along.
- Most frequently used marketing tool for small agencies.
- Can generate more clients and referrals than any other form of advertising.
- Versatile — easy, quick, inexpensive to tailor for different niches.
- Expected — exchanging cards is an established business practice.
- Creates name recognition, personalizes you and builds credibility for your agency.

Avoid these 10 Common Business Card Mistakes

Don't produce a business card that:

1. Does not clearly define what you do.
2. Does not serve as a "memory hook."
3. Projects a bad image of your agency — is tacky or cheap.
4. Does not act as a marketing tool.
5. Appears cluttered and messy or has type too small to read.
6. Contains non-essential information.
7. Is out-of-date — contains old information.
8. Does not use the space on the back of the card.
9. Is not professionally printed.
10. Is printed on thin card stock.

What goes on your card?

The basics — your logo, your business name, address, phone, fax, e-mail and web site addresses, and then individual names and titles. If it is short enough, you can include your Unique Selling Proposition as well as the services you provide.

No room, you say? You can always build on a very valuable piece of "real estate" that is often left vacant — *use the back of the card!* It costs very little more to print on the back, but this can increase your response rate by *ten times*. If you use the back, you *can* tell your clients all the services you provide.

On the back you can also put important phone numbers, i.e. hospitals, police, fire, pharmacy, etc. This will increase the chances of your prospects and clients putting it in their wallets or purses. This will help increase your referrals!

Production Tips

Professional-looking business cards are a small cost compared to the cost of losing prospective clients because of an unprofessional image.

- **Have them professionally designed and printed.** Your image is everything.
- **Use the best paper available.**
- **Stay away from larger printed cards** that tear easily. They look unprofessional and will make your clients think that your agency is unprofessional. Instead use 3" x 2 1/2" cards — they fit nicely into business card holders, wallets, etc.
- **Choose easy-to-read typefaces** that are just large enough so that your clients can read them. Use no less than 12 pt. Typeface, especially when marketing to the elderly market.

- **Proofread, proofread, proofread.** Have everyone OK his or her individual card before it goes to press. There is nothing more disheartening (or more common!) than finding that the fax number is incorrect, or the e-mail address is missing a letter, or that your director of nursing — Mary Shulz — is misspelled as Shultz…

Where do you hand your cards out?

Hand them out wherever you can — hospitals, senior housing, local grocery markets, etc. Hand them out with brochures. (Include two — one for the recipient, and one for referral.)

SAMPLE OF BUSINESS CARD

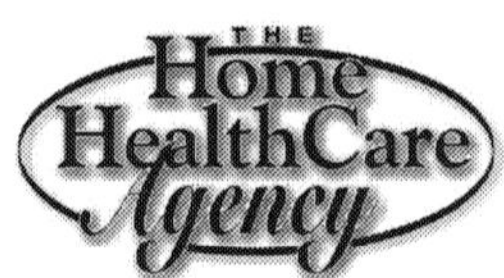

Jane Anne Doe R.N.
Nursing Supervisor

Professionals Caring For People at Home!

123 Anystreet • Anytown,AB 65432
Phone: (555) 123-4567 • Fax: (555) 123-7654
www.thehomecareagency.com

FRONT: 80% OF ORIGINAL SIZE

Services We Provide

- Nursing
- Homemaking Service
- Medical Equipment
- Pediatric Care
- Hospice Care

Call Us Today for a FREE In-Home Assessment

BACK: 80% OF ORIGINAL SIZE

CHAPTER NINETEEN

Yellow Pages Advertising

Develop advertising as good as the product.

— Leo Burnett

After several years of spending thousands of dollars on yellow page ads, we decided to work with The Real Yellow Pages marketing department and conduct a marketing study. We wanted to determine the cost-effectiveness of Yellow Pages ads on increasing calls. We *specifically* wanted to measure the effectiveness of using various sizes colors, copy points, pictures, and placements in the Yellow Pages.

Here is a summary of our findings:

- Color ads increased our "hits" by over 40%.
- Placing the ads under Nurses as well as under another heading such as Home Health or Home Care Services increased calls by 30%.
- Pictures did help in attracting inquiries.
- Larger ads had a greater response rate.
- Including copy (information about our company) increased response.

Other important facts we determined from our research:

- A person who uses the Yellow Pages to select a Home Care company is usually a family member dealing with a crisis, or a patient who requires help at home.
- Most of the people using the Yellow Pages had never used or required the services of a Home Care company and they needed information and help to understand "how the system works." They were looking for ways to help them make the correct choice. Other than price, they did not know how to differentiate one agency from another.
- If your company has never advertised and your "brand name" is not well known, it is important to differentiate yourself in the Yellow Pages ad.
- Many people use their logo in bold, large print on the Yellow Pages ad instead of a *strong headline*. It is more effective to state in bold type *why* someone should call your company over another. Advertise benefits, benefits, and more benefits in your headline!

I strongly recommend that you have your Yellow Pages ad professionally designed. Do not rely on Yellow Pages to come up with an exciting attentiongrabber ad. They are in the business of filling pages and selling ad space — not graphic design and marketing.

HERE ARE SOME EXAMPLES OF SUCCESSFUL YELLOW PAGE ADS. YOU DECIDE.

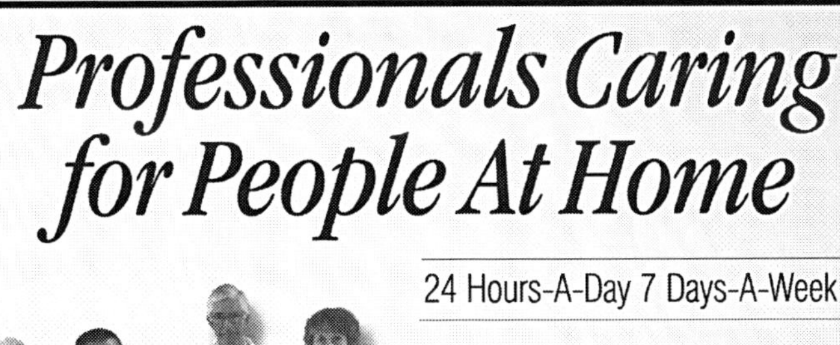

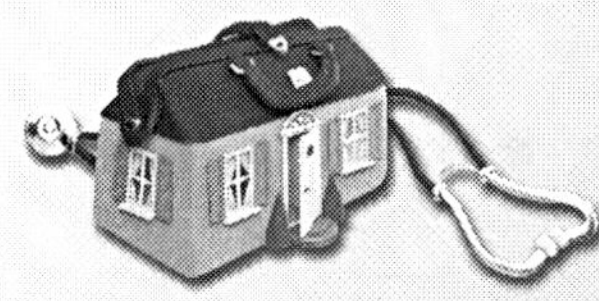

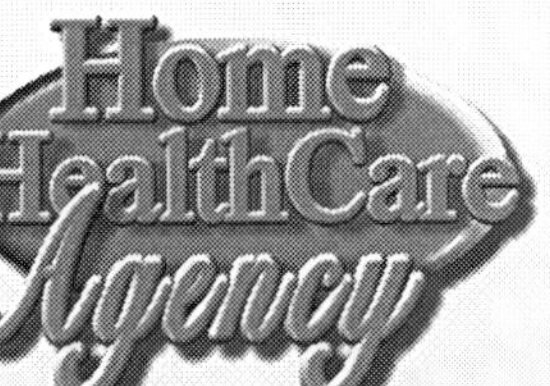

EXAMPLES OF SUCCESSFUL YELLOW PAGE ADS...CONTINUED

Now, You or Your Loved One Can
Go On Living at Home . . .
Our caregivers and customized care plans can help you remain in the comfort and security of your own home when you need assistance, instead of a nursing home.
The Home HealthCare Agency is one of the nation's leading providers of comprehensive home health services to private individuals, case managers, insurance companies, health maintenance organizations, third-party administrators, nursing home and hospitals.
Our Services include:
• Skilled Nursing
• Home health Aides
• Physical Therapy
• Occupational Therapy
• Speech Therapy
• Medical Social Services
• Sitters and Companions
• Private Duty Services
To talk to one of our Case Managers in your area, call us today:
1-800-555-1234
Call Us Today for a
FREE In-Home Assessment
Visit Our Website!
www.thehomehealthcareagency.com
Home HealthCare Agency
Quality Care in Your Own Home Guaranteed!
Please call our Free Recorded message to learn more about our agency and services we provide. 1-800-555-5555

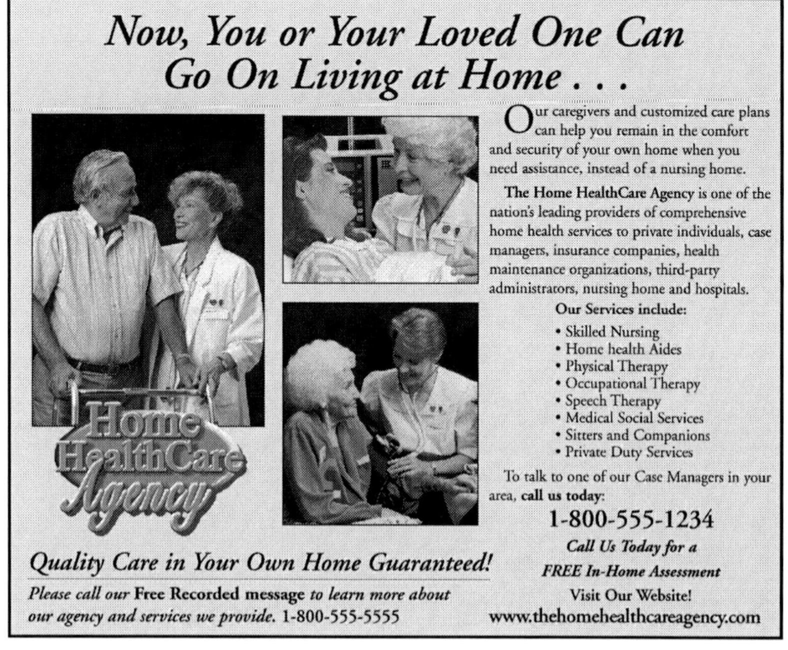

Responding to Inquiries

Equally important as the appearance of your ad is the way your staff handle the calls from Yellow Pages ad inquiries. If you want proof, call various companies in your Yellow Pages book. Ask about services for your parent and evaluate how you are treated and how helpful other companies are when *you* call.

Most Home Care companies have not invested in training their staff on telephone manners and salesmanship. Many potential sales are lost because staff members are not equipped to handle calls.

Years ago, I answered the phone in one of our branch offices and the caller, an elderly gentleman, said he found our number in the Yellow Pages. He wanted to know how long the company had been in business and wanted me to tell him why our company was "better than any of the other home care companies." I responded to his *perfectly legitimate questions*, explaining that we were a small company, owned by a nurse and that we prided ourselves in providing personal attention to each of our clients.

He then told me he wanted to arrange private duty in-home help for his wife and wanted to have someone come out to their home and discuss services. He insisted that since we provided personal attention, *I* should make the in-home visit myself. I *did* make this visit and when he discovered that I was the owner and founder of the company, he was impressed that I came rather than send someone else to make the visit. The outcome of that decision turned out to be very significant to my business. We had only been in business for a year and we were struggling to get off the ground.

This client did arrange to have private duty for his wife, and then eventually additional care for himself. We provided services to this couple for *ten years*. The couple lived in a private seniors apartment and became one of the best referral sources we ever had. He liked to tell people about his call to our office and how "the president of the company made a house call!"

My point in telling you this story is that our Yellow Pages ad initiated the call — personal attention and providing information *made the sale*.

By the way, this client spent over $100,000 a year for 10 years on our services.

Yellow Pages do work.

Remember:

1. Use an attention-getting headline — advertise benefits!
2. Make the prospective client want what you are offering.
3. Tell them to call you.
4. Prepare a plan to train your staff on handling inquiries and track the source of the calls.
5. Follow-up and ensure that your ads are conveying accurate information.
6. Use a professional to design your ads. Keep the ads clean, uncluttered and professional looking.

CHAPTER TWENTY

Brochures & Collaterals

We cannot direct the wind,
but we can adjust the sails.

— Unknown

Brochures and collateral pieces (folders, information sheets, specific care pamphlets, any printed materials that you pass out) are advertising materials that tell a bigger story than your business card or a sales letter. It is a printed piece that serves as an "identity piece" as well as a direct sales tool.

Your Company's Brochure

Your company brochure is your primary "collateral" piece. It should serve as a marketing tool that provides a detailed description of your agency, your services, testimonials, philosophy of agency, community involvement, etc. It is a very important part of the selling process.

Your brochure should be used as an introductory marketing tool that gets you one step closer to your prospect. It serves as a non-intrusive means for your prospects to pre-qualify your agency without having to meet with someone from your agency. Your brochure may not close the sale on its own, but it will introduce a prospect to your agency and open the lines of communication between you and your prospect.

What Should a Brochure Say?

Start with a healthy headline. The headline should be catchy and express a benefit to the client. It should contain specific words that your target market will identify with.

For example: *"Now Dad can go on living at home… and I can stop worrying."*

Your brochure should list *benefits* — not just features. Explain what your client will receive for his/her money — how much value they will receive, how they will feel better, live longer, regain independence, and enjoy freedom, happiness and companionship.

Include testimonials from satisfied clients and use high quality color photographs. Include your Guarantee!

General Production Notes

Brochures can be designed in various sizes depending on your message and budget. They come in single sheet 8 1/2" x 11", 8 1/2" x 14" or multisheet booklet formats. "Single sheet" brochures can be folded any number of ways. You're most familiar with the tri-panel format (bi-fold, often *called* a tri-fold, though it has only two folds). However, there are other options, depending on the flow of your copy and the overall look you want. Your printer can show you gate folds, tri-folds and accordion folds. *The fold is part of the design.* It determines how your client opens your brochure, what she reads first, where her eyes go, etc.

When including color illustrations and photographs, I recommend that you print on coated paper such as gloss or a very nice matte. This will give you the most professional-looking results.

Don't cut costs on the design of your brochure. If you are operating on a low budget and have planned for a lengthy brochure with lots of text, then I would suggest that you reduce the amount of text in your brochure, and spend less on the printing and more on the design. A well-designed, concisely written brochure is always more successful than a lengthy brochure that appears unprofessional.

Tips for Successful Brochures

- **Keep it glossy and colorful.** Your brochure should be a professional looking printed piece. It is not a letter! Include photographs and color illustrations or graphics. Choose a bright, quality coated paper. Color and a coated paper says "High Quality." Some people will only purchase services they believe are high quality, reliable, etc.
- **Stress the benefits your services offer.** Clients want services to help them maintain independence and stay involved in the world around them. It is important that they feel in control of their lives, so offer choices to make them feel appreciated.
- **Address the interests and specific concerns of the audience** for each particular brochure, i.e. widowhood, care giving, grandparenting, etc.

- **Use short, clearly worded sentences** and avoid industry jargon such as NAHC, HCFA, PPO, etc.
- **Use a reader-friendly 12-point type (font),** especially if most of your clients are senior citizens. Allow space between the lines and use paragraphs with clean headings, illustrations and photographs.
- **Keep the brochure looking and reading personal.** Write in the first person (We, or I).
- **Don't put timely information** (dates, one-time events, references to current events) on the brochure. Don't date your brochure by saying that your business is 5 years old; say that you have been in business since 1996. (This is a date that's OK to put!) This will prevent you from having to reprint your brochure every year.
- **Use bulleted lists and bold face copy** to identify important points.

How to use a brochure effectively.

Your brochure is *part* of the process of building a relationship with a potential client. Use it to introduce your agency, inform prospects of your agency's services, educate them about new concepts, and help to get the appointment to close the sale.

Send brochures to prospects who are "pre-qualified." A brochure should always be sent to a new prospect that your agency has already talked with or has been referred by someone you know. *Always include a sales letter.*

Brochures can also be sent to a broader mailing of prospects — but only if their names are on a well-researched list of a specific demographic group that would consider your services (senior citizens, rehabilitation patients, doctors and medical administrators, etc.). Attach a personal cover letter with your brochure saying who you are and the reason for sending your brochure to them.

Another recommendation is to get an endorsed letter from a happy client (church group, trust officers, hospital administrators, etc.). This concept is simple: The "endorser" provides letters *on his letterhead* to people who know and trust *him*, but do not yet know *you*. The letter serves as a general endorsement, recommendation and/or introduction of your company — and is accompanied, of course, with one of your brochures. Ideally, the mailing is done using the endorser's letterhead envelopes and not your own.

The endorsed mailing is the only form of mailing to get 100% opened and 100% read. Endorsed mailings are powerful because of the increased readership and the credibility you gain from the endorser.

A Final Note: Don't rely on your brochure alone to build relationships with prospects. A brochure will not usually close a sale — your prospect and future client will need personal contact. But your brochure can open that door, if it presents your image and services well.

SAMPLE BROCHURE

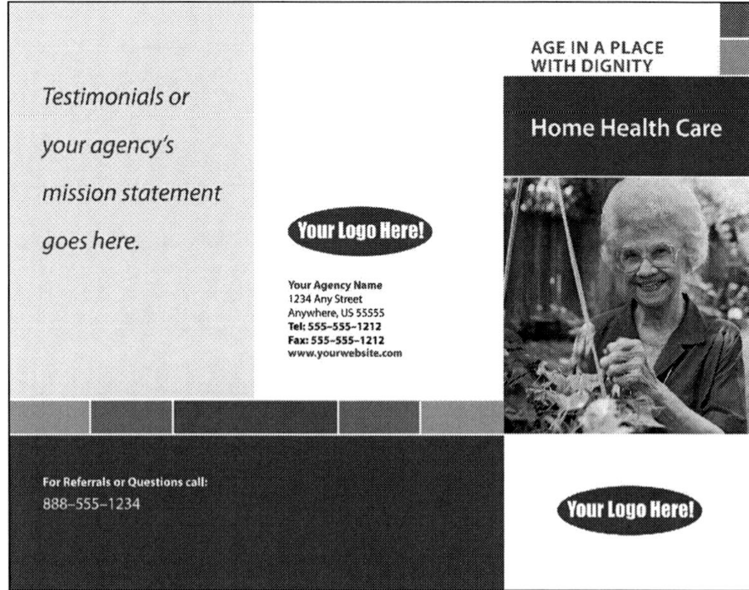

OUTSIDE: 35% OF ORIGINAL SIZE

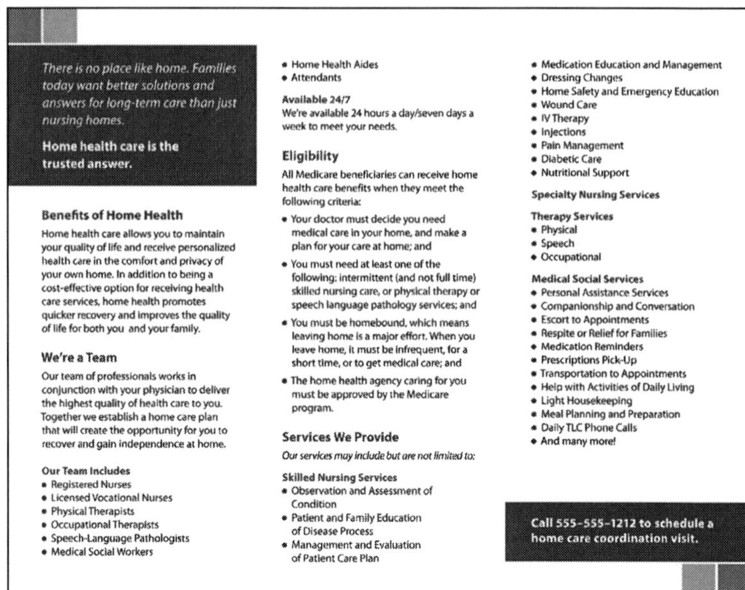

INSIDE: 35% OF ORIGINAL SIZE

CHAPTER TWENTY-ONE

Direct Mail

If you miss seven balls out of ten, you're batting three hundred, and that's good enough for the Hall of Fame. You can't score if you keep the bat on your shoulder.

— Walter B. Wriston

Direct mail is one of the most powerful ways to market your Home Care company. Direct mail marketing refers to directly-mailed advertisements/offers, mail orders, coupon advertising, postcard offers, even offers on a web site. It encompasses any method of marketing that attempts to make a sale *right there and then to the prospective client.* Direct mail doesn't always make the sale, but it can produce lists of crucial leads that result in sales.

Advantages of Direct Mail over other advertising methods are:

1. You can more accurately measure and test results.
2. You can concentrate on a target audience.
3. You can personalize your marketing.
4. You can expect a greater overall number of responses.
5. You can enjoy repeat sales from former clients and obtain referrals.

Why Direct Mail Often Fails

1. The company has no direct mail expertise.
2. The sales letter is poorly written.
3. The mailing list is not appropriate for the offer.
4. The list itself is inaccurate and does not reflect the desired demographic and/or it was not current.
5. The "offer" is not strong enough to elicit a response from intended target audience.

How to Make Direct Mail Work

Use the right list.

- This is the most important element. It must reflect the group you are targeting and it must be up-to-date.
- Lists that you might consider for your business to include: seniors with disposable income living in houses or apartments, 45–65 year-old children of seniors, physicians, case managers, lawyers, and trust officers. (see "who influences Home Care Buying Decisions" — Chapter Four — diagram for more examples of direct mail)
- You can purchase lists from list brokers. You will need to be specific about your demographic and area. Ask how current the list is.
- Make sure the list broker can supply you the list in the computer program you need — will you be printing labels off a computer in your office? Will you use an outside print house to print up individualized envelopes? Will you be using a mailing house? All may have different programming requirements.

- You can compile your own lists over time, but this will need to become a conscientious effort — probably assigned as a side task to someone on your team.

Get them to open the envelope!

- If the direct mail piece looks like junk mail, it will become junked mail. You don't want to go so far as to mislead the recipient, but you want him to open the envelope.
- Think of clever, snappy, intriguing words or images (sometimes a classy, formal look is effective) to put on the outside of the piece that will ensure it is opened.
- If your mailing is not large (500 or less) the best way to ensure that a direct mail piece will be opened is to *hand address the envelopes*. Gather the team and go at it. This takes a while — but you get responses. Everyone opens a letter addressed by hand! Think about it… *Don't you?*
- Avoid having a "bulk mail" look. Avoid tell-tale cursive typefaces that *try* to look like handwritten addresses. These are a give-away that this is a mass-mailing. It's better to use a plain typeface for the addressee and look formal than to look phony.

Include a letter.

- Letters almost always out-pull mailing packages without a letter.
- Home Care companies should spend some intensive hours in research before they write the first direct mail letter. Ask some current clients what they like about doing business with you and begin your letter with those benefits.
- Write about your clients' needs and problems. List the solutions you can provide to those problems and benefits that you offer.

- Include testimonials from satisfied clients. Testimonials improve response rates!
- Emphasize your unique services. (Available twenty-four hours a day, seven days a week, homemaker services, informative newsletters, etc.)
- Tell why your staff is special, i.e. carefully selected, screened, referenced, experienced, extensively trained, bonded, supervised, in uniforms, highest paid.
- Your letter must then invite them — convince them! — to take action on the offer.

Design your piece for maximum impact.

- Your headline must get attention. Your headline is really an ad for your sales letter. Ask for action in the headline of your brochure or letter. Get your reader interested.
- Blue is a good second color, but red ink with black generally gets the best response. Don't over-use red — use it primarily for highlights.
- Use short words, short sentences, and short paragraphs. Use large print for seniors.

Have an irresistible offer.

- The offer may be in the letter itself, with no other printed piece in the envelope — or the offer may be printed up as a separate piece that accompanies the letter.
- You must make your offer enticing. The better the offer the better the response. Create a desire. Make your reader really want what you are offering.

Make the reader take action.

- Structure your offer in such a way that you will get a response.
- You must have a deadline. If you don't have an expiration date you will not have direct response.

Make it easy for the recipient to take action.

- Include a pre-addressed, pre-paid envelope if the offer is a mail-back response.
- If you want them to call, give them a real name to ask for.

Keep good records.

- If you are testing multiple markets, include a code on your coupon/offer/mail-back card that will enable you to log response results from different mailings and/or offers.
- Send a test mailing and measure the results. A few dozen or a few hundred letters will give you a good feeling for the response you can expect.
- Log your responses daily.
- Log the repeat business you get from the initial respondents to truly measure the value of that initiating direct mail campaign/offer.
- Analyze your data and plan your projections for the next campaign so that you earn the maximum profit.

Some Direct Mail Offer Ideas

1. Coupons for a variety of services: foot care, house cleaning, etc. Note: Research shows that seniors, in particular, appreciate and use coupons
2. Drawing for a year of flower delivery (one bouquet a month)
3. One free overnight "patient-sitting"
4. A day of free homemaking services for seniors who have just lost a spouse.
5. New Mother Care gift certificates
6. Free newsletter for seniors

I hope you will try direct mail if it is at all feasible for your business. Your competitors may not have tried it, which may give you a chance at broader exposure in your market. Plus, you can get a head start on this major marketing method of the future.

The following is a list of brokers to help you with your mailing list:

- SRDS (Standard Rate and Data Service catalog) found at your local library.
- Best Mailing Lists (demographic compiled lists) 1–800–NYC–BEST
- Act One Mailing Lists (demographic compiled lists) 1–800–ACT–LIST

SAMPLE DIRECT MAIL BROCHURE

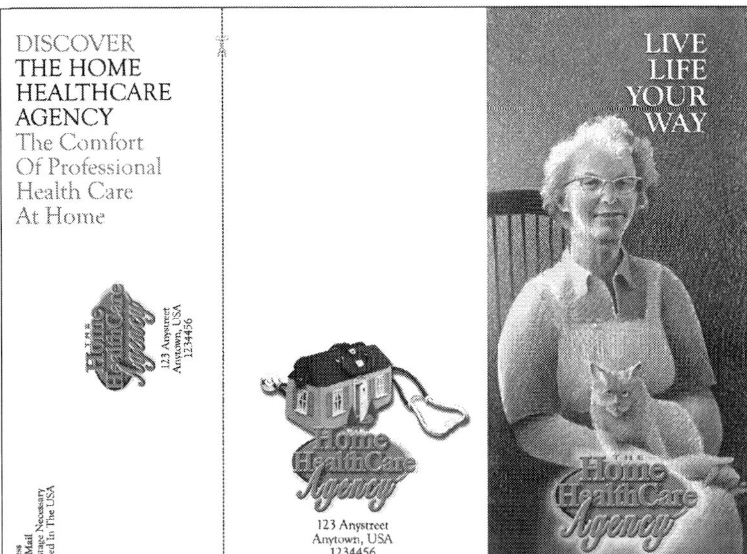

OUTSIDE: 35% OF ORIGINAL SIZE

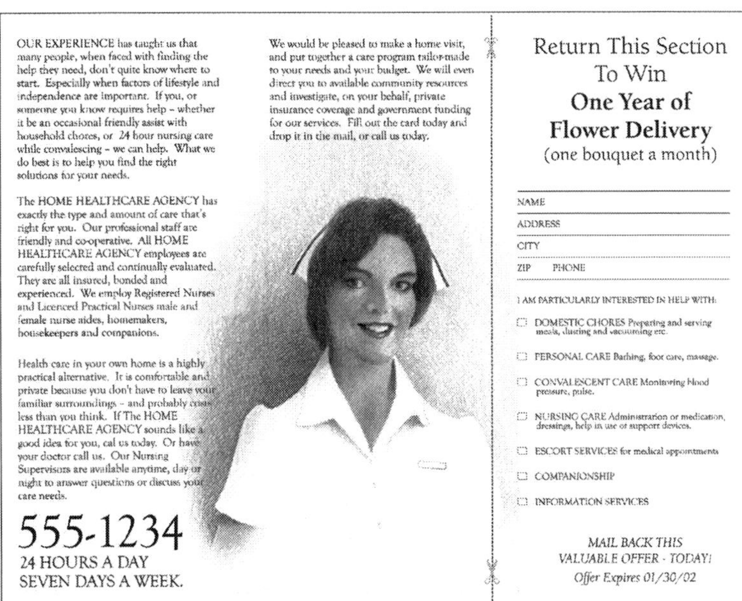

INSIDE: 35% OF ORIGINAL SIZE

SAMPLE DIRECT MAIL POSTCARD

BACK: 50% OF ORIGINAL SIZE

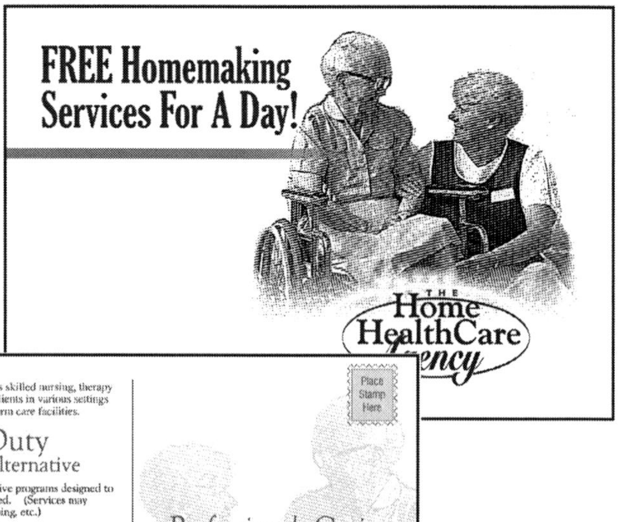

Place Stamp Here

The Home HealthCare Agency provides skilled nursing, therapy services and personal care services to clients in various settings including private residences and long term care facilities.

Private Duty
An Affordable Alternative

We are experienced in delivering effective programs designed to provide seniors with assistance they need. (Services may include meals, bathing, light housekeeping, etc.)

How It Works

Whether you are living at home, apartment, or seniors' residence, our services can be tailored to your individual needs and will enable you to purchase a few hours of service per day up to 24 hours of care seven days a week depending on your needs.

Our employees are carefully selected professionals with years of experience. Each is insured and supervised.

Please call us Today to schedule your FREE Day of Homemaking Services

615-555-1234

Offer Expires 1/9/01

Professionals Caring For People At Home!

THE
Home
HealthCare
Agency

123 Anystreet • Anytown,AB 654321
Phone: (555) 123-4567 • Fax: (555) 123-7654
www.thehomecareagency.com

FRONT: 50% OF ORIGINAL SIZE

CHAPTER TWENTY-TWO

Newspaper Advertising

The best way to have a good idea is to have a lot of ideas.

— Dr. Linus Pauling

Demographics and Readership of the Newspaper

Newspapers are read by approximately 18% of the adult population. In addition, nearly half of all adults receive home delivery of a Sunday or weekend paper. Two thirds of adults read the newspaper on an average Sunday. The most faithful readers are aged 45 to 54 (who are 29 percent more likely than average to be heavy newspaper readers), and those aged 55 to 64 (who are 22 percent more likely). — Kim Long, The American Forecaster Almanac, 1993 Business Edition.

Advantages of Newspapers

There are many advantages to advertising in newspapers. For Home Care companies, these include market coverage, positive consumer attitudes and flexibility.

- **Market Coverage**
  An obvious asset to newspaper advertising is the extensive market coverage your business can receive. When your agency wants to reach a local or regional market, newspapers offer an extremely cost efficient vehicle.

- **Positive Consumer Attitudes**
  Your prospects maintain positive attitudes toward newspapers in general. Readers generally perceive newspapers — including the advertisements — to be very accessible, current, and highly credible sources of information.

- **Flexibility**
  One of a newspaper's major strengths is that it offers great geographic flexibility. Your company can choose to advertise in some markets and not in others. Newspapers are often flexible in the actual production of the ads as well. Unusual ad sizes, full color ads and inserts are some options available.

Disadvantages of the Newspaper

Newspaper advertising also has some disadvantages. These include: short life span, clutter, limited coverage of certain groups, service criteria and poor reproduction.

- **Short Life Span**
  Although a great many people do read newspapers, they read them quickly and they read them only once.
  The average life span of a daily newspaper is only 24 hours.

- **Clutter**
  A high clutter factor is a serious problem with most newspapers. This is particularly true on Sundays, when information overload reduces the impact of your company's advertisement.

- **Limited Coverage of Certain Groups**
  Although newspapers have wide market coverage, certain market groups are not frequent readers. For example, newspapers traditionally have not reached a large segment of the elderly or those speaking a foreign language — and both groups are potential prospect for your Home Care company.

- **Service Criteria**
  Consumers seeking immediate Home Care services primarily do not use the newspaper to find this type of service. Therefore, your ad must be informative and stress the benefits of your services in order to catch the attention of those who may have a need for your services at a later time.

- **Poor Reproduction**
  The reproduction quality of newspapers is comparatively poor and limiting, especially for color advertisements. The speed necessary to compose a daily newspaper prevents the detailed preparation and care in production that is possible when time pressures are not so great. The actual newsprint paper is porous and gray. Unless the color ad is produced by someone who understands newspaper print quality, newsprint can make color ads look muddy and very unattractive.

Approach Print Advertising with the Right Mindset

Advertising is nothing more than salesmanship in print. Most companies try to do cutesy ads and they try to do institutional ads. An institutional ad is one that tells people how great and wonderful their company is (not their benefits — just their company) and tends to keep the company name in the spotlight instead of the needs of the reader. For the most part, these ads are a waste of time and money.

People don't actually care about how great *you* are. They care about the caregiver service and benefits that your agency offers that others don't. How are you going to improve the quality and value of *their* lives? How are you going to make their lives easier? These are the questions that your prospects want answered in your advertisements.

Your ads should be created to stimulate a direct response — immediate actions. Few companies truly understand the purpose or reason for running newspaper ads. It's to stimulate a direct and immediate response — either a qualified inquiry, phone call or request for an in-home assessment — or better yet to get a new client. Ads are expensive so they better work fast!

The purpose of newspaper and magazine advertising is to get new clients. But, it is not the clients that you get from the newspaper that will make your business profitable. It's the referrals that you get from the new clients. Referrals are the primary reason you advertise. Referrals are less expensive and can lead to compounded profits for your agency. I strongly suggest that you have a solid referral system in place before you start advertising in the newspaper. (See the chapters on Referrals in Part III.)

The Anatomy of a Great Ad

The Headline

The headline is the most important component of your ad. Nearly six times as many people read the headline as the body copy of an ad. The #1 purpose of a headline is to point the reader to a "reward" in your body copy. Give them a reason to read your ad. The wrong headline (or having no headline) can result in the failure of the ad to accomplish its primary goal: to lead the reader into the body of the ad. Use your best headline — one that provides the reader a benefit.

When you have decided on your headline, you have created 80% of the effectiveness of your ad. Never settle on one headline without testing at least five or ten. Never consider running an ad without a headline. Write five to ten headlines and have your colleagues pick the best one and use it.

If you have time, you can test headlines more thoroughly through split run testing. Split run testing is when you choose two or three of your best headlines and run them simultaneously in various publications to see which one gives you the best response. To differentiate each headline you can provide a different offer for each headline, have a different phone line designated for each headline or assign each ad containing a different headline a code number for the prospect to provide you when inquiring about your offer in the advertisement.

Develop the headline so it appeals to your prospect's self interest. Promise the prospect a big, big benefit in the headline — one of your company's most dominant benefits.

Once you've found the best headline, try it with different body copy. Then, when you've found the best most effective headline and copy, test different offers and call-to-action approaches in your ads.

Improving each component of your ad raises your return that much more. So keep improving your ad until you achieve the results you want.

The Body

Your prospects will only go on to read the body copy if the headline arouses their interest. Your body copy should be written in first person direct: i.e. "We give you the very best care, when you need it!"

Long copy or short copy? The universal perception that people won't read long copy is false. Ads are either boring or interesting. If your copy is interesting, your prospects will spend the time to read your ad whether it is a half page, full page, or multiple pages. Write as much as it takes to make your case, whether it takes one paragraph or two pages.

In your body copy, include information, education and useful information to the reader. Write your copy in human language and stay away from using technical medical jargon. Use short words, short sentences, short paragraphs, bullets and personal copy. Tell your prospects the benefits of your services; explain how your agency will help them.

The Call to Action

Check the ads in the newspaper, isn't it amazing how many agencies stop short of asking you to take any specific action? Too often, even if they do ask you to "Call today," they give no really good reason, incentive, or reward for calling.

You don't want to look like so many of the ads out there — ads that your competition may be running — that have no headline, look very institutional, contain little or no copy, with no call to action. Here are the mandatory ingredients of a call to action:

1. Tell them exactly WHAT you want them to do.
   i.e. *"Use our homemaking services coupon."*
2. Tell them exactly HOW you want them to do it.
   i.e. *"Call us today."*
3. Tell them exactly WHEN you want them to do it.
   i.e. *"Before your coupon expires."*
4. Give them clear incentive to ACT.
   i.e. *"Save X amount on homemaking services if you act now."*

Images in Ads

Illustrations (photos, line art, special graphics, etc.) often take up quite a bit of space in your ads, thus they should work just as hard as your headlines to sell your services. An art/graphic element should illustrate the same promise that you make in your headline. Your illustrations must arouse your prospect's curiosity. He or she must glance at the photograph, identify with it and be compelled to read the body copy of your ad.

Our research has shown that photographs "sell" more than drawings. They attract more readers. They are better remembered and they sell more services. Photographs represent reality, whereas drawings represent fantasy, which is less believable. Ads with photographs are twice as memorable, on average, when they are printed in color.

Ten Basic Rules about Newspaper and Magazine Advertising

1. Have a strong catchy headline to gain the attention of readers.
2. Tell something newsworthy — the ad should contain important, useful information about the services you provide.
3. Make a free offer — don't try to hard-sell anything in the newspaper. Offer a free brochure about your Home Care services or a free home assessment but don't try to sell per se.
4. Keep your illustrations/art as simple as possible with the focus of interest on one person. Crowd scenes don't pull.
5. Don't show human faces enlarged bigger than life. They seem to repel readers.
6. Ads in four-color cost 50 percent more than black-and-white, but on the average, they are 100 percent more memorable. A great bargain!
7. Use a serif font/typeface (This is a serif font. **This is not: this is a san-serif font.**) for the body copy of your ads. The little flourishes on the ends of letters that are called "serifs" make the words easier to read. San-serif typeface can be harder on the eye, especially if it is in one copy block.
8. When writing body copy for your ad, keep it interesting. You can't bore someone into using your services — you can only interest them into using your services. Write your copy as if you are writing to a friend. Keep it first person singular or plural (I, we) or second person (you). Use short sentences and short paragraphs, and avoid using difficult words.

9. Include testimonials in your ads. Readers find the endorsements of fellow clients more persuasive than taking your company's "word for it."

10. Bigger is better! Bigger ads pull better than smaller ads.

Where should the ad go?

If has often been said that the three most important factors in choosing investment real estate are (1) Location (2) Location (3) Location. A similar guide can be used when running your ads in the newspaper. Namely, the three most important factors are (1) Position (2) Position and (3) Position!

The #1 reason people don't respond to a newspaper ad is because they don't see it!

You are probably thinking that running your ad in the Lifestyle section on a right-hand page is the best place, right? This is not necessarily true!

As soon as your prospective clients sit down to read their daily newspaper, they immediately divide it into sections. A man may ask his wife for the Sports section, the wife may ask for the Food section. Their kids may ask for the Comics. Business people may want the Business section. Others may pick up the Society pages. And so on.

But very few people read the entire paper. In fact, most people read no more than two or three sections.
Think about it — *do you?*

What does all this mean? This means that the very best place for your company's ad to appear for maximum visibility and readerships is on the *front page of a section.*

And the second best place? *The back page of a section.* Why? Because even though most people don't read (or even open up) every section, most people at least touch every section. They may touch it for no other reason than to pass it to someone else or to pick it up to throw it out. And, while they are handling each section, they are extremely likely to look at the front and back pages of those sections.

While they are glancing at those pages, if they happen to see an eyecatching ad — an ad with a "killer" headline or illustration — they just might stop and read that ad to see what it is all about.

So, know this: Your #1 job is not to get your prospect to *read* your ad. It is to get them to *see* your ad!

An ad that appears on the inside of the business pages will be seen by everyone — everyone, that is, who reads the business section, and that's it! However, if your ad appears on the front or back of any section, it will be seen not only by business people but also by almost everyone who handles the paper! Yes?

#1 secret of running effective ads in the newspaper is:
Run your ad on the front or back of a section!

Buying Space

Buying space at the right price is just as important as presenting the right message through your marketing materials. (Sometimes even more important!) The greatest service, offer, and ad copy in the world will not overcome bad economics, and one way to suffer bad economics is to over-pay for ad space.

When using a new publication for the first time, you must lean on them for their very best rate. Negotiate hard. The media representative may try to force you into "frequency commitments" in order to grant discounts, but I recommend not doing this before you test your ads.

Ask your representative about buying "remnants" (available space not yet sold shortly before run date). If you purchase remnant space you'll need to have ads ready to place with little notice.

Do not let your agency be pressured into a high-priced space under any circumstances. At the same time, don't ever get upset and burn the bridge with a publication just because you can't get the discount that you want. I recommend ending your negotiation with something like: "I'm sorry we can't do business this time. I will have to use my ad budget in other publications. If you have a last-minute cancellation or remnant, please contact me." Keep your door open.

The publication may not counter your offer immediately. As they see your ad placed in other publications, they'll come back to you — guaranteed!

No matter how well your company does with your advertising, avoid revealing to the publication how well you are doing, especially to the representative who sells you discounted space. Being humble and not bragging about your success can be most profitable!

Here is the Ultimate Secret when placing your ad in the newspaper to save your company a ton of money!

When placing your display or recruitment ads in your local, regional, state, trade, or any other publication, *you can often dictate the rate that you will pay for placing your ad.*

First, obtain the publication's rate card or rate information and discount the amount of the ad space by 30–50%. Second, send the publication your "camera ready" ad, a check for the amount *you* have figured. Include a letter explaining your request inviting them to either hold the ad and check for up to X amount of days — as a "stand-by" to fill a remnant (open space available) or last minute cancellation — or to return the check and decline the insertion order.

The psychology: A check in the hand with a ready-to-print ad is worth two "in the mail." Your ads will find their way into the publication.

This is one of the biggest kept secrets. Try it, and save a bundle on your newspaper advertising.

Seven Limitations of Small Ads

1. Small ads don't impress your prospects as much as large ads.
2. You can't use copy to tell your prospects about your services.
3. You can't use color in small ads. It would be too expensive.
4. You can't include an illustration in your ad to draw readers.

5. You can't create a large volume of sales quickly.
6. You can't create the impression of importance of your services like you can with a large ad.
7. You can't get the best positions for your small ads in newspapers.

Seven Advantages of Small Ads

1. You can run a whole series of small ads for the price of a single full page. Thus, small ads enable your company to advertise frequently at low cost.
2. If your company offers a variety of services, you can feature a different service in each ad in a series of small ads.
3. Instead of running a series of pages in a single newspaper, you can advertise in multiple newspapers or publications by using small ads.
4. You can gain flexibility by putting part of your ad budget into running big ads and part into running small ads.
5. You can offer free booklets, literature and brochures about your services.
6. You can get special paid position where only a small ad would fit — such as running your Home Care services ad alongside a special medical health editorial or feature.
7. Great for limited advertising budget! Lets your company get in the paper.

Analyzing the Results from Your Ads

Some questions you need to ask of your ads are:

- What caused one ad to pull better than another? Headline? Offer?
- What incentive did you put in the ad to compel your prospect to take action?
- How much did a lead or project cost? How much did it cost per sale? How many sales did you generate? (Review Chapter 17, "Track Your Results.")
- How many prospects converted to new clients?

You must analyze your ads — what they say, how they say it, the headline, whether they present your USP, the offer, the action you direct your prospect to take, the costs and the resulting sales. After your analysis tells you which offer, headline and copy works best, try to improve upon your ads.

Testing your Ads

Take your best most effective ad and begin testing different versions (start with headline) against each other. Changing a headline could out-pull another 10 to 1. Once you've got the best-pulling headline based on quantitative analysis, try to improve the clarity and appeal of the offer and rework the copy if necessary. Test different offers and guarantees.

Test one variable at a time. It means isolating the variable so you are positive of the source of the different results. For example, if you are changing the headline, don't change the offer. If you're comparing the guarantee against another, don't change the headline.

Keep accurate track of each response and its results: inquiry, new client or previous client. Keep track of every piece of information pertaining to your ads. Then, when you have all the results logged for each ad or each different variable that you tested, compare the results and use the better one. Then keep testing until you are satisfied with your results. (See Marketing Tracking Sheet in Chapter 17.)

SAMPLE OF SUCCESSFUL NEWSPAPER AD

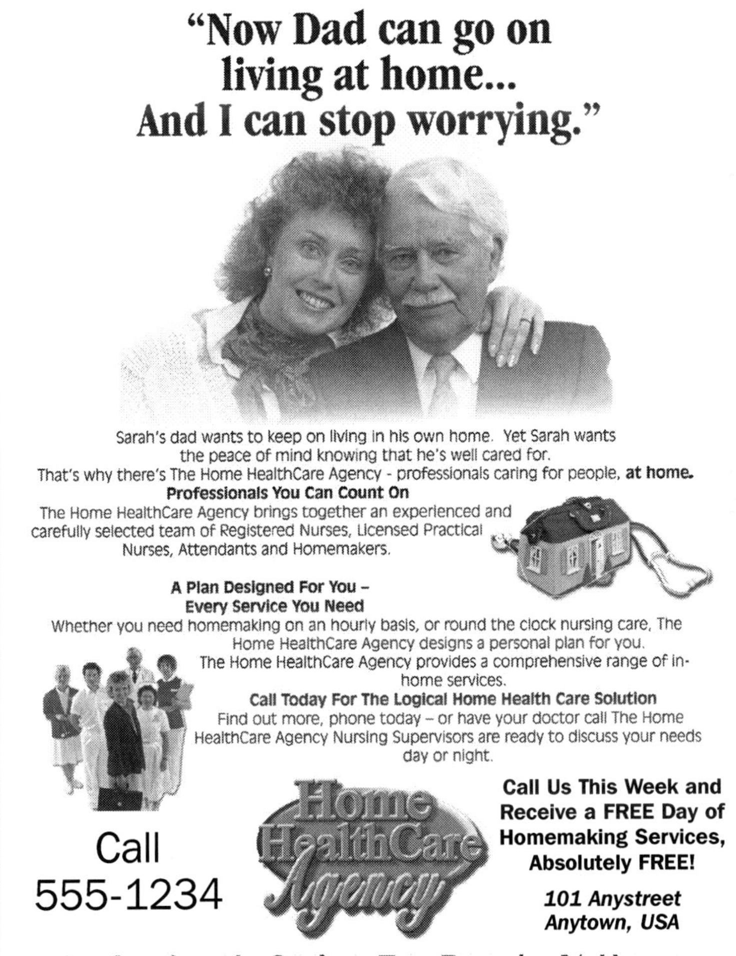

"Now Dad can go on living at home... And I can stop worrying."

Sarah's dad wants to keep on living in his own home. Yet Sarah wants the peace of mind knowing that he's well cared for.
That's why there's The Home HealthCare Agency - professionals caring for people, **at home.**

Professionals You Can Count On

The Home HealthCare Agency brings together an experienced and carefully selected team of Registered Nurses, Licensed Practical Nurses, Attendants and Homemakers.

A Plan Designed For You – Every Service You Need

Whether you need homemaking on an hourly basis, or round the clock nursing care, The Home HealthCare Agency designs a personal plan for you.
The Home HealthCare Agency provides a comprehensive range of in-home services.

Call Today For The Logical Home Health Care Solution

Find out more, phone today – or have your doctor call The Home HealthCare Agency Nursing Supervisors are ready to discuss your needs day or night.

Home HealthCare Agency

Call
555-1234

Call Us This Week and Receive a FREE Day of Homemaking Services, Absolutely FREE!

101 Anystreet
Anytown, USA

Professionals Caring For People At Home

SAMPLE OF SUCCESSFUL NEWSPAPER AD...CONTINUED

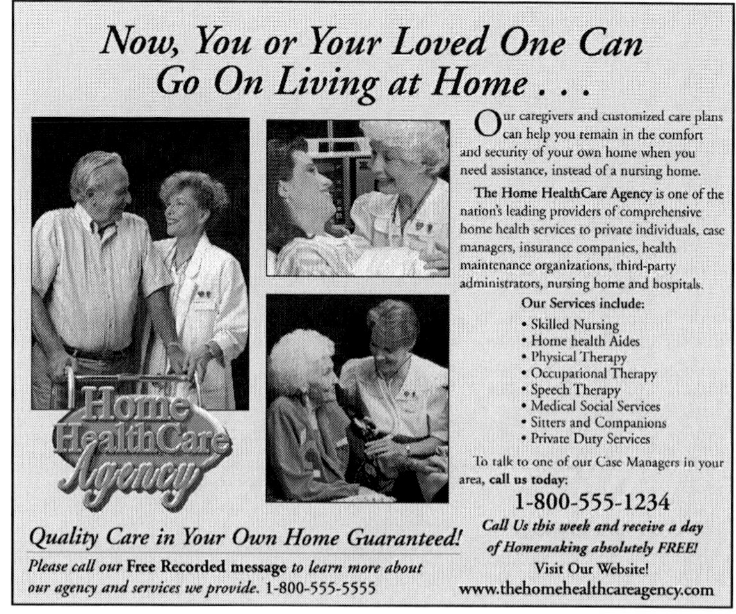

Effective Ads Can Run for Years.

Once you have perfected your ads and they are pulling effectively and generating profits for your company, your ads can run unchanged for years in the same market (and sometimes even a different market) and be successful for your company without diminishing returns.

When running an ad, remember that your target audience is always new clients. Existing clients using your services are not going to read your ads. They have already read and decided to use your service. Always address your ad to the unconverted prospect.

An ad should be dropped only when you can come up with another ad that is more successful. Remember, you are advertising to a "passive parade," not a standing army. New prospects are seeing it all the time as they move in and out of your market. *You* may see your ad every time, but your prospects may only see it once or twice out of five runs. So if you have a winning ad, keep it!

Remember these five basic concepts when writing your ads.

1. Command attention from your prospect.
2. Show prospects the advantage of using your service.
3. Prove that what your company is advertising has that advantage.
4. Persuade people to believe that advantage.
5. Make a call to action.

Good advertising is salesmanship multiplied! Put your sales presentation into your ads and you have multiplied your sales staff thousands of times over. Follow these principles and sit back and reap profits your company never thought possible.

CHAPTER TWENTY-THREE

Billboard and Signage Advertising

To be heard from afar, bang your gong on a hilltop.

— Chinese Proverb

Billboards and other Signage advertising can be extremely beneficial for your company if used properly.

Advantages of Billboard Advertising

- **Inexpensive**
  Outdoor advertising is one of the least expensive of all the major advertising media based on cost per thousand (CPM).
- **Long life**
  Billboards are great for messages that need to be repeated. An audience sees it numerous times over a long period of time.

- **High impact due to size**
  Billboards are big, colorful, hard to ignore, larger than life — and difficult to miss!
- **High market selectivity**
  Billboards can be placed in a specific location that will reach your target audience more readily.

Disadvantages of Billboard Advertising

- **Creative limitations**
  The message must be simple and brief. You can't develop an involved story or copy points.
- **Viewer has many distractions**
  The viewer is usually traveling in a car. There is a greater chance that the viewer's attention will be disrupted by traffic or other advertisements — this prevents him from viewing your ad.
- **High level of criticism**
  Some critics feel that outdoor advertising is visual pollution.
- **Limited availability**
  Criticism of outdoor advertising has led some areas to restrict or ban billboards.
- **Short exposure per viewing**
  The average person is exposed to an outdoor message for only a few seconds.

SAMPLE BILLBOARD

"Now Dad can go on living at home...
And I can stop worrying."

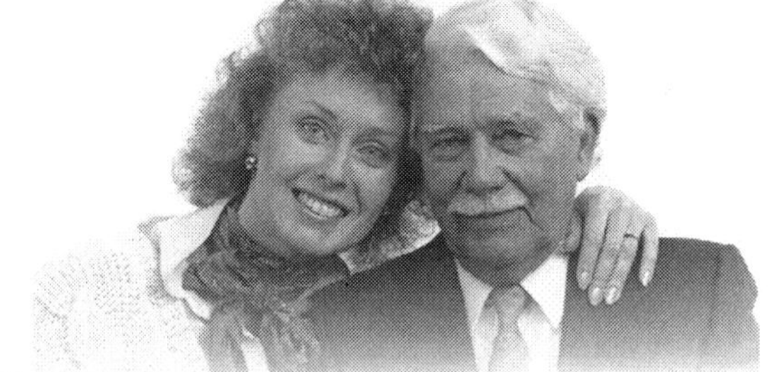

THE HOME HEALTHCARE AGENCY
"Professionals Caring For People At Home"

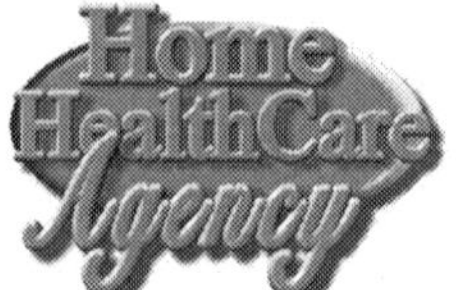

Call Us Today
for your FREE In-Home Assessment

555-1234

Types of Billboards

There are many different styles and sizes of billboards and signs from which to choose, depending on the audience you are trying to reach and the size of your agency's budget. The most common outdoor/indoor billboards and signs include:

- Painted Bulletin — outdoor (size: 14' x 48')
- Poster Panel — outdoor (size: 9.7' x 21.7' or 10.5' x 22.8')
- Bus Shelter Signage — outdoor
- Subway Signage — outdoor
- Station Poster — indoor (train, bus, subway stations, air terminals)

- Car Cards — indoor (inside bus, trains and subway cars)
- Posters — indoor (elevators, washrooms)
- Exterior Ad-carrying sign — on exterior of buses and taxis

Sign and Billboard Placement

Placing your billboard or sign in the right location is probably the most important decision you'll make — other than the design and message.

Your primary target audiences are going to be:

- Seniors between the ages of 65–85
- Children of seniors between the ages of 45–65
- New staff recruits who on average will be between the ages of 25–45

In order to maximize your advertising dollars, your agency must place your sign or billboard in the best locations to reach the greatest number of your target audience.

Seniors between the ages of 65–85.

You are going to get the highest success rate by placing your billboards where this target audience is most apt to be. We have had tremendous success reaching seniors by placing billboards in the following locations.

- **Bus Shelters and Benches**
  These are great locations because seniors often use city transit for their only means of traveling. Place on routes going to hospitals and shopping malls.

- **Senior Community elevators — 8.5" x 11" Posters.** These inform the senior of the services that your agency provides along with contact information to receive a free brochure.

- **Buses, Trains and Subway Cars — interior Car Cards** Place on routes going to hospitals and shopping centers. Car Cards allow your agency to have a longer message describing the services and benefits available to the senior along with contact information. You have their attention for an average of 20–30 minutes so your message can be more involved. Some car cards let you include "tear-off" or "take-one" sheets. If they do, be sure to include your contact information for a free brochure or consultation. This will increase your response rate ten times.

Children of seniors between the ages of 45–65

For this target audience, I recommend the following locations for the greatest success rate.

- **Interstate Locations and along high commute routes** Billboard Poster Panels are great for reaching this audience because of their high level of commuting. I also recommend that you place your billboard along hospital and shopping mall routes. These routes are traveled by a high number of people in your target audience.

- **Air, Train, Subway, Bus Terminals** Station Posters are very successful in reaching your target audience due to their locations. Because your target audience travels frequently and uses air, train, and subways on their commute, these station posters catch their attention.

- **External Ad-carrying Signs** Another effective means of advertisement your agency can use is to buy space on an external ad-carrying sign located on buses and taxis. Because of this audience's high level of commuting, your chance of reaching them with your message via this style is very high.

New staff recruits, ages of 25–45

I recommend using the following billboard placements and styles:

- **High Traffic Areas**
  Near hospitals and shopping centers Billboards (Panel Posters) along the route corridor are effective.
- **Bus Shelters and Benches**
  Place signage at ad-carrying Bus Shelters and on benches. Place them on bus routes that go to hospitals and shopping centers.
- **Inside Buses, Trains and Subways**
  Use Car Cards on routes that go to hospitals and shopping centers.
- **External Ad-carrying Sign**
  Great to place on buses and taxis that travel in high traffic areas and/or on hospital and shopping center routes.

Ten Tips for Designing a Great Billboard Advertisement

Effective outdoor billboards require a strong creative concept that can be instantly understood. Your idea needs to be creative because your message has to get attention and be remembered by your audience. Most importantly, your billboard has to make a point quickly.

1. Have it professionally designed.
2. Have a strong creative concept that is instantly understood.

3. Keep your copy to a minimum for outdoor signs. Keep words and sentences short, using catchy phrases. *Note:* Interior Billboards and Posters have a more aptive audience and can contain longer copy with a more involved sales message.

4. For your layout, use a simple "visual path." Begin with a strong graphic, followed by a catchy headline and end with product/brand identification.

5. Graphics and illustration should be an eye-opener. Get your billboard noticed.

6. Use bold, bright colors and have strong contrasts. For example, use dark colors against white or yellow. Yellow often provides contrast and has a greater impact to an audience.

7. Your background should never compete with your message in the foreground.

8. Keep type easy to read — especially for Panel Poster bill-boards. Most of your audience will be in motion while viewing your billboard. Avoid using "all-capital" letters or ornamental scripts. These are too hard to read. Use simple, clear, uncluttered type for best results.

9. Include your Brand Identification. Don't forget to include your logo and/or positioning statement (when there is room and "reading time") along with contact information on your billboard.

10. For Painted Bulletins and Poster Panel Billboards, design for distance. Reading distance is an important consider-ation in designing and planning outdoor signage. Professional advertisers will know the correct viewing scales. (See Tip #1!)

CHAPTER TWENTY-FOUR

Radio Advertising

Don't be afraid to be amazing.

— Andy Irwin

Radio is the most personal and intimate of all media. For many of your target audience listeners, it functions as a good friend — particularly for seniors. Radio has one great advantage over print media, and that is *the human voice.*

Radio advertising is a great marketing vehicle for your agency to reach multiple target markets successfully and inexpensively. Our success with radio advertising was two-fold — as a publicity generator and as an advertising medium.

When we started our agency, we sent press releases to many of the local radio stations that had older listening audiences. We were guests on one of the local talk radio shows talking about our new services. These approaches were extremely successful for our agency and this was free publicity — and therefore free advertising! These forms of publicity are discussed in Part III of your manual (Chapter 44 — Radio and TV Talk Shows). In this chapter we'll look at using Radio as a medium for purchased advertising.

Our Home Care agency also placed ads with local radio stations to advertise our agency's services to the local community. We purchased 30-second slots in both morning and lunch hours, targeting the 45–65 and 65–85 audiences. Our message included our services, the benefits of choosing our agency, how to apply for care, how care is paid for, and the merits of our qualified and screened staff. We ended with a "call to action."

Some of our ads featured dialogue between a grown child and an elderly parent discussing the options and convenience of using our services. A line that we found to be extremely successful (and often repeated) was: *"If you or somebody you know requires help at home, we can help you find the care you need. Call us today for a free brochure or in-home consultation."*

This one sentence consistently attracted the attention of many listeners who were in need of home care services or knew of someone who did. It resulted in an amazing number of new clients and referrals.

Advantages of Radio Advertising

- **Target Audiences**
  One of the most important advantages of radio advertising is that it allows your agency to reach its specific target audience through specialized programming. For example, many stations feature talk shows that specifically target seniors. Sometimes the host of the show is a senior and/or the show provides information about community activities, health concerns, and senior-related topics.

- **High Flexibility**
  Of all the media, radio has the shortest closing period — the period between purchasing and actually placing your ad. This means that in many cases, copy for your ad can be submitted up to airtime. This flexibility allows your agency to

quickly adjust your ad for current news events. For example, if there is a seniors community activity coming up, your agency might alter some of the copy at the end of your existing ad to announce that you will be sponsoring the event. You might suggest that folks visit your display booth to receive a free brochure or promotional item.

- **Inexpensive**
  Radio is probably the least expensive of all media. Because airtime costs are relatively low, extensive repetition of your advertisement is possible. In addition, the actual pre-air cost of producing a radio ad is low, especially if the local station announcer reads your message on air, bypassing recording costs.

- **High Level of Acceptance**
  Radio has a high level of acceptance at the local level. Your target audience has favorite radio stations and local radio personalities, which they listen to regularly. Messages delivered on these stations — and messages read by these personalities — are more likely to be accepted and retained.

Disadvantages of Radio Advertising

- **Message has Short Life**
  Unless your ad is repeated frequently, it will be missed or forgotten by your target audience.

- **Lack of Visuals**
  Radio obviously prevents the use of visuals. This limits the amount of "activity" you can have in your ad.

- **Clutter**
  The large number of radio stations, combined with frequent repetition of ads, has created an enormous amount of clutter in radio advertising.

Seven Tips for Creating a Great Radio Commercial

1. **Identify your agency's name early in the commercial.**
2. **Identify your agency's name often in the commercial.** To help the listener remember your agency, your ad must mention your agency's name at least 3 times during a 30-second commercial and at least 5 times during a 60-second commercial. And since the last thing your audience hears is what they will often remember longest, I recommend mentioning your agency's name at the very end of your commercial.
3. **Promise the listener a benefit early in the commercial.** Early in the commercial, tell your target audience the #1 benefit they will receive from using your services. "Giving you the freedom to live your life in your own home" worked great for us.
4. **Keep your ad simple.** Radio is great for building brand awareness for your agency but it's a poor medium for using long lists of copy points. Give your target audience one or two important benefits at a time in a conversational style approach. This method will bring you greater results!
5. **Make your ad informative.** With minimal words, tell your audience the services your agency provides, how qualified your staff members are, how you screen your staff, how your audience can apply for services, how they can qualify, etc.

6. **Have a senior radio personality read your ad.**
   If there is a senior radio talk show personality whom seniors enjoy listening to, I recommend having that person read the copy for some of your ads. This will benefit you because your target audience already knows and trusts this person, which will give your message greater credibility. You can either have the commercials pre-recorded (which will ad to your costs, but will give you greater placement flexibility) or your ad can be announcer-read each time on air.

7. **Offer something FREE!**
   Always offer your audience a free home care services brochure, free in-home consultation, or something to make them take immediate action to call your agency.

CHAPTER TWENTY-FIVE

Television Advertising

Think big, believe big, act big,
and the results will be big.

— Unknown

Television Advertising is an extremely valuable marketing tool for many businesses that are selling a tangible product with a national market and who have huge marketing budgets. I am not saying that television advertising won't get you new clients — because it will. But at what cost? Our experience from trial and error, (and losing a lot of money from television advertising) supports our recommendation to your Home Care agency to forgo television advertising. It may gain some market share, but is not the most efficient or best use of your marketing dollars to get clients.

Having advised this, I still suggest that you read this chapter and consider your unique business situation when developing your overall advertising plan. Local stations may very well provide a good outlet for you, especially if you can advertise on a local health issue talk show with a wide enough viewership.

If you are absolutely set on having a television ad, I recommend that you consider the following to increase your commercial's success rate.

- Have a celebrity endorse your agency. This can be a local celebrity but it should be someone who is fairly well known in your area. It's better if the celebrity has used your services (for themselves or for their family members) and really is happy with your agency.
- Budget $100,000-$150,000 for television advertising.
- If you personally appear in your own ad, you must be prepared that you'll become recognized. Anyone who is on TV becomes a minicelebrity. People will recognize you — especially if your TV advertisement is effective and runs often.

Advantages of Television Advertising

- **Show and tell**
  You can show a creative demonstration of your services.
- **Geographic market selectivity**
  You can reach a local or national audience.
- **Create impact on viewer**
  Television uses sight, sound, color and emotion — and therefore a greater level of client involvement. Exposure on TV can make your service appear more important, exciting and interesting to youraudience.
- **Influential**
  People have a greater tendency to believe companies that advertise on television because it has become such a primary entertainment and information source for our culture.

Disadvantages of Television Advertising

- **Expensive**
  Although the "cost per viewer" is low, the overall cost for your agency to produce and continue to run your commercial is extremely expensive, especially if your agency is small or midsize.

- **Clutter**
  Television suffers from a high level of commercial clutter. Your ad must compete with others in a short time period and your "message" has a great chance of being forgotten or missed completely by your audience.

- **Nonselective audience**
  Although the networks attempt to profile viewers, their descriptions are quite general, offering your agency little assurance that the appropriate audience will be viewing your commercial. Thus TV advertising includes a great deal of waste coverage — communication directed at an inappropriate (and often uninterested) audience.

- **Inflexibility**
  Television also suffers from a lack of flexibility in scheduling. Most network television is bought a year in advance, which leaves your agency with only limited time slots available. In addition, it is difficult to make last minute adjustments in terms of scheduling, copy or visuals, as compared to other marketing media.

- **Perishable ad message**
  Unless your agency runs your TV ad on a consistent advertising schedule, your message will be forgotten very quickly.

How to Make TV Commercials that Sell

The same rules apply to developing a great TV ad that apply to developing any great ad; but there are three strategies that I recommend your agency consider when developing your TV ad.

Slice of Life/Demonstrations

This technique involves portraying a "real life" situation that your target audience can identify with. For example: A scene with your Home Care nurse caring for a senior in their home, illustrating that your services provide the senior/client with a better quality of life. Your target audience will immediately identify the value of your services which is intended to lead to an inquiry or a new client. If you choose to use the "slice of life" approach, be sure to keep your scenarios "real" so that your target audience will relate and identify a need for them.

Testimonials

Using testimonials, which show loyal clients testifying to your agency's virtues, can be very successful. A good example is to have a scene with one of your existing clients telling one of his/her friends just how helpful, great and convenient it is to have your agency caring for them. When using loyal clients to testify, avoid those who would give such polished performances that your target audience would think they were professional actors. The more amateurish the performance, the more credible.

Problem Solution

This technique — creating a problem, agitating the user and solving the problem with your service — is as old as television but is still extremely successful. For this technique I recommend that you show a senior or a family member having a problem caring for him or herself or their parents. For example: A scene of the mature daughter of an elderly parent discussing with her husband that she does not have enough time to care for her parent. Next scene: A nurse assisting the elderly parent, with the daughter saying to the audience something like "I'm sure glad I can rely on the Home Care Agency. They have provided my mother with the care she needs and at the same time eliminated my worries about my mother." This technique is effective because it speaks directly to the emotions and sentiments of your target audience.

Three tips to use when developing your TV Commercial

1. **Brand Identification**
   Use the name of your agency within the first 10 seconds of your commercial. When you first start advertising on TV, you have to keep reinforcing your agency's name throughout your entire commercial to up the audience "recall" factor.

2. **Show your service in action.**
   The more helpful your services look in your commercial the more you will sell. People need to see the benefits!

3. **Grab the receiver's attention.**
   Your commercial is short so you must grab the viewer's attention immediately within the first frame. For example, the first scene could show a senior in need of immediate assistance — with one of your nurses coming to his aid. This would immediately grab the attention of your audience.

CHAPTER TWENTY-SIX

Website Presence

You can't sit on the lid of progress.
If you do, you will be blown to pieces.
— Henry J. Kaiser

A Website is a powerful new marketing tool that can serve as a great equalizer: Your agency has the opportunity to reach the same universe of potential business as larger national agencies for a fraction of the cost.

Benefits to You

- Reduces cost of sale
- More information can be provided to your client without having to tie up staff
- Pre-qualifies prospects
- Inexpensive — can change content regularly with minimal cost
- Provides detailed information — more than any other single medium — through pictures, video, sound, text and links to related sites

- Can get prospects' names and e-mail addresses
- Faster — can post up-to-date information for your clients and prospects
- Interactive — can get feedback from clients and prospects
- International — can reach remote clients and prospects who may be traveling or moving to your area, or who may be looking for care for their parents
- 24-hour medium — you can send and receive information any time
- Creates a sense of community with your clients — through chat rooms, discussion groups, newsletters — can strengthen relationships with clients

Benefits to Your Prospects

- Access in the comfort of their own home
- Not pressured to make a decision
- Access from a remote/long distance location
- Saves time
- Provides comprehensive information about your company

The Internet as a Marketing Tool

The Internet is one of the most useful yet over-hyped marketing opportunities. There has been a widely-held misperception, not only by the Home Care Industry but also by every industry, that "if we build it they will come." This is not entirely true. In order to attract prospects to visit your website, it must be interesting and provide them with some kind of valuable information that will make them revisit *and* tell others about your site. The following are a couple of tested, proven and almost universally valuable uses of your website:

First, have your website be a client-services, education, and information center. Don't focus on it as being a client-acquisition source. For example, just by having a FAQ's page (Frequently Asked Questions) on you website — with clear, detailed answers to these questions — you can reduce the number of inquiry calls to your office by fifty percent. This will free up your staff to do other money-making sales activities instead of answering questions that could be answered by visiting your website.

Second, begin asking for, collecting and organizing the e-mail addresses of visitors to your site. With this list, your agency can do virtually free, push-button marketing anytime you like. Your agency can send out your newsletter or other important/useful information to your clients and prospects.

Ten Reasons to Put Your Business on the Internet

1. **The Internet is the fastest growing marketing medium in the world.**
   The Internet currently has about seventy million people online globally with that number expected to grow to over seven hundred million over the next few years.

2. **Take advantage of remote marketing.**
   The Internet allows your agency to expand your sales and marketing reach into the emerging global marketplace. Through your website, prospects and their family members living in remote, even international locations, can learn about your services as well as keep in constant contact with your agency for virtually no cost.

3. **Compete with larger national agencies.**
   The Internet can serve as a great equalizer for your agency when competing against large national agencies. Your agency has the opportunity to provide better, more useful

health care information, and other specialized features which can give your agency an advantage over your larger competitors.

4. **Showcase your professionalism and image.**
   Prospects will be impressed with your agency's "forward looking" vision and will feel more comfortable about receiving services from you.

5. **Offer 24-hour service.**
   By having a website, you allow prospects and their families to contact you or get questions answered twenty-four hours a day, seven days a week, 365 days a year. This is an obvious competitive advantage for an agency.

6. **Allow feedback from clients.**
   Unlike with conventional advertising media such as brochures and newsletters, Internet sites allow your agency to request and receive feedback from clients at no extra expense.

7. **Serve your local market.**
   Whether your agency is located in New York City or Jackson Hole, there are probably enough local prospects with Internet access to make it beneficial for your agency to consider web marketing.

8. **Post job opportunities.**
   A website is a great tool for finding great employees. Finding qualified employees is often the hardest part of running a successful agency. Use the Internet to broaden your search and outreach to find the brightest employees.

9. **Because your competition is not on the Internet.**
   If your competition has not yet developed a website, this is a great opportunity to jump ahead of the crowd and be known as the innovative and service-oriented agency to prospects.

10. **Increase sales.**
    There are over seventy million people on the Internet. Almost all the people visiting your website are specifically looking for information about Home Care services. This can create a much higher percentage of sales for your agency.

If you want people to use your services, you've got to sell — and a very big part of selling (perhaps the biggest part) is keeping in touch with people over time. Repetition breeds sales. Gentle persistence is the key to selling. Most prospects are simply not ready to buy right away, so if you have a website strategy that says: "We'll sell them the first time they visit," you're missing at least ninety-five percent of the business you *could* be getting. The only way your agency can be "gently persistent" with a website visitor is to:

- Sell your prospect on the idea of giving you his/her e-mail address.
- Follow-up intelligently.

How do you get people's e-mail addresses?

The only surefire way to do this is to *ask*. I recommend that your website have a "guest book" or some type of registration that visitors can fill out. Make it easy for them to sign up. Don't have a large form to fill out. Ask many times, putting the offer to register on multiple pages as links. The more times you ask, the more times they will say yes.

Give them a reason to sign up. Offering to contact them with new information and updates to the site are both good reasons. Whatever is your offer, keep it interesting and let them know about it. *Reassure them that you are not going to sell or share the list with anyone.* If you are going to have a "guest book," then you need to be up front about why you have it. Tell them something like this, for instance:

If you'd like updates of new site materials — such as newsletters and industry and health related news — please give us your e-mail address and we'll add you to our announcement list.

Your website should be about offering information — lots of it, adding to it all the time. It's not about scanning in your brochure and letting it sit there, static indefinitely. You can do that if you want to, but don't expect to get good results.

I recommend having regular news to report: new services, new client success stories and other interesting news that will make people come back to visit.

Rules for Maximizing the Value of Your Clients and Prospects with E-mail

1. Mail as often as you can.

2. Only mail when you have something worthwhile to say. If you combine rule number one and two, it comes down to this: you can mail as often as you like as long as it is something worthwhile and interesting to the prospect/client.

3. Keep your e-mail short — just give them the facts and tell them what to do next.

4. Make it easy for people to get off the list. They should be able to send you a simple e-mail that is sufficient for you to take them off the list right away. At the end of all e-mails that you send out, briefly repeat the procedure for them to be removed from your list. This is common courtesy.

5. As long as you are making it easy for them to take themselves off the list, let them know that it is fine with your agency if they share the e-mail with their friends/families and make it easy for these people to join the list, too. Word-of-mouth advertising is always the best advertising and you can encourage it.

Eight Keys to an Effective Website

These key characteristics help define an effective website and I recommend that you use as many of these in your website as possible.

1. **Your site must be appealing, so have it professionally designed.** It should be inviting and informative, with constant re-invention.

2. **Your site must be valuable, useful and fun.** It should be immediately useful, giving prospects reasons to bookmark it.

3. **Your site must be current and timely.** The content should appear fresh, giving prospects reasons to come back.

4. **Your site must be easy to find and use.** Your site should be widely registered and have well-chosen key words.

5. **Your site must have user-friendly on-page navigation.** It should have easy-to-follow on-page hyperlinks.

6. **Your site must involve the visitor.** It should invite the visitor to come in, register and stay awhile.

7. **Your site must be responsive to users.** It should be open and responsive to visitors' suggestions and comments. It should encourage visitors to provide feedback. If your agency is located in an area with large segments of Spanish or Asian people, then having a multi-language site might be beneficial for your agency.

8. **You site must load quickly.** Include interesting graphics, but don't overload your site with so many complex elements that it takes a long time to download.

Seven Ways to Use Your Website to Market On-line

1. **Give away advice.** Giving away free Health Care-related advice to various interest groups and prospects allows your agency to build relationships and increase conversion rate with prospective clients.

2. **Use links.** Having hyperlinks can be a great benefit to you. With one click on a word or graphic, your prospective client can move to another area of your site for information about a particular service or feature your agency offers. In addition, you can have links to other sites that your clients and prospects might tend to go to regularly, i.e. pharmacy, weather sites, etc. This adds value to your site, encouraging more visits.

   Another way to use links is to have other sites provide links to your site. For example, your community might have a seniors website that could include a link on their site that takes seniors directly to your site. This is a great marketing tool because you are endorsed by a credible referral source to seniors.

3. **Encourage bookmarks.** Bookmarking is a way of recording or indexing your website for future reference. Tell your prospects on your first page — as well as on other pages — to bookmark your site so that they can get back easily the next time they log onto the internet.

4. **Maintain fresh content.** If you aren't constantly adding new links, articles, and information, your website will become old news. Keep it updated!

5. **Be included on directory listings.** A great way to have prospects locate your website is to have your site listed in the many directories and indexes. Some directories,

like Yahoo, are great search engines to help your prospects find your website. To learn more about getting listed, visit www.searchenginewatch.com

6. **Select the right key words.** Most directories and search engines look for key words. It is important that you think in terms of the prospect. What are they going to be looking for? How can you help them find your site? For example, even if prospects know that you are ABC Care, they won't necessarily know the name of your site so you must get listed with key words such as: Home Care, Health Care, Senior Care, etc., to better help them find your site.

7. **Have an on-line newsletter.** An e-mailed newsletter is a great way to keep in touch and build relationships with your clients and prospects. It is a way to give people a sample of your expertise and philosophy. A friendly newsletter lets them become familiar with your agency, and makes it easy for them to reply. Start by asking existing clients and prospects to sign up to receive your letters and then ask them for referrals or ask them to refer others to your site.

One last bit — or byte

You should be clear about your intentions before you invest the time and money to establish a presence on the Internet. Many large companies spend thousands of dollars on the development of their websites. As a small company, you can't afford to make an investment and not get a return on this investment. The good news is that by combining traditional marketing methods with some high-tech techniques, your website can do more than stand as a bits and bytes version of your paper marketing materials.

Don't let the Internet take away from your commitment to more reliable, predictable marketing tools. Do get on the Internet and move at a comfortable speed. A website is a great addition to your existing marketing mix and one that can be extremely profitable if you follow the proven techniques and advice provided in this section. Good luck and have fun surfing!

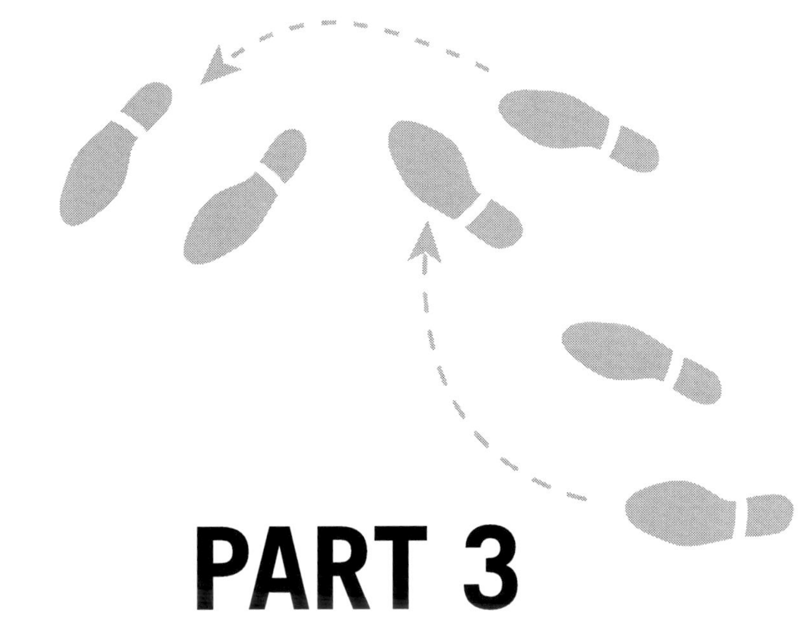

PART 3

Marketing Does Not End After the Ads Run…

CHAPTER TWENTY-SEVEN

Internal Marketing

Good teams become great ones when the members trust each other enough to surrender the me for the we.

— Phil Jackson

For Home Care companies, the caregivers cannot be separated from the service.

The caregiver is a significant part of the medical service. In reality, the clients "buy" the people when they buy a service — and service is often a labor-intensive performance. In labor-intensive service firms especially, the quality of the employees influences the quality of service, which in turn influences the effectiveness of service marketing.

Home Care companies must practice internal marketing successfully and they must market to their own employees and to employee prospects creatively and aggressively.

What is Internal Marketing?

Internal marketing is attracting, developing, motivating, and retaining qualified employees through job-products that satisfy their needs. *Internal marketing is the "philosophy" of treating employees as clients.*

The ultimate goals are to encourage effective marketing behavior and to build an organization of marketers willing and able to create true clients of the employees. A knowledgeable, satisfied employee is your best marketing agent. In essence, internal marketing is to *treat your employees the way you want them to treat your clients!!*

Competing for Staff

Hiring the best possible staff to perform services is a key factor in services marketing. The Home Care industry has a tremendous challenge of recruiting and retaining both clinical and non-clinical staff.

Given the current shortage of health care workers — especially nurses — this problem is likely to get worse. If ever there was a time for Home Care companies to compete more effectively for talent, that time is now. The entire service sector (not just the health care industry) is experiencing a labor force shortfall that will intensify in the years ahead. There are simply not enough qualified employment candidates to satisfy the service sector's appetite in the next ten years and beyond.

The Home Care companies that use their marketing know-how to shop the labor market will fare best in the future.

Recommendations:

- Use multiple methods.
- Cast a wide net.
- Do not lower hiring standards.
- Use recruiting methods other than classified ads, but when you run an ad, make it creative and track the results.
- Use career fairs and recruit-an-employee programs with finder fees.
- Offer flexibility in work hours and flexible benefits.
- A note on the future work force: *Rigid thinking will not work.*

If you do not recruit, orientate and retain qualified workers, it will not matter how much money you spend on marketing and how many new clients you get — you will not be able to fill client requests.

Offer a Vision

A paycheck may keep a person on the job physically, but it will not keep a person on the job emotionally.

Caregivers, especially home care caregivers, need to know how their work fits in the broader scheme of business operations, and how their work contributes to the company. They need to have a “cause” because serving others is just too demanding and frustrating to be done well each day without one.

Home Care companies have to stand for something worthwhile and they must communicate this vision to employees with passion.

Visions should be simple, and communicated at every opportunity and communicated personally by top management.

The company's vision should also be communicated in training and orientation manuals, employee handbooks, newsletters, and through employee incentive plans.

A common mistake that is made by some Home Care companies is to provide a one-week orientation course and an annual workshop — then consider employees "trained." Turnover in Home Care can be a direct result of employees not feeling competent, confident or motivated to perform services.

What you can do to be different

Home Care companies need to help existing middle managers and supervisors become better teachers. Home Care companies must change their mindset with respect to employee education:

- from provider orientation to a client orientation
- from employees being replaceable to employees being *irreplaceable*
- from reactive to proactive

Emphasize Team Play

People want to identify with a group, to make a contribution, to express themselves, and exercise creativity. They want to feel good about their jobs, because this makes them feel good about themselves.

One of the best ways to create a feeling of camaraderie is to have monthly meetings for all shifts, and quarterly meetings for all employees. These meetings need to be upbeat, informative, and supportive. At these meetings, you can announce employees of the month, new service developments, humorous experiences, and emphasize the team nature of the company.

Creating a Team Atmosphere will greatly improve morale. Home Care service is demanding — frequently frustrating and stressful. It is common for home health providers to be so stressed that they become less caring, less sensitive, less eager to please. What clients perceive as *impersonal* behavior is often the *coping* behavior of weary servers who have endured much stress in their roles as caregivers.

When employees feel isolated, just "doing their one job," their job performance suffers, their job satisfaction level suffers, the client does not receive the very best care, and your business will ultimately suffer. Therefore, it is imperative that you maintain a positive team atmosphere with an understanding of the difficulties and stress that Home Care inherently brings. Talk it out, share, compare notes, and as a unit come up with solutions. Think as a team.

Measure and Reward

The goals of internal marketing will not be met if employee performance is not measured and rewarded.

Employees need to know that they will be measured on how well they do and that it is worthwhile to do well.

Dollar rewards and incentive bonuses for hours worked, longevity, and satisfactory performance evaluations are important. But these factors are not the only ones to consider when determining rewards.

A few suggestions on rewards:

- *Link employee rewards to the company's vision and strategy.* Reward employee performance that supports the company's vision and business plan.

- *Distinguish between competence pay* (compensation for doing one's job) *and performance pay* (extra rewards for outstanding performance).
- *Use multiple methods to reward outstanding performers*, including financial rewards, non-financial recognition, and career advancement. For senior management, also consider the possibility of rewarding employees with stock and making them owners.
- *Remember the power of saying "thank you."* Rewards do not have to be expensive — the sincerity of the recognition is most important.
- *Develop enduring reward systems* and use short-term programs such as bonuses for meeting company objectives.
- *Stress the positive.* Use reward systems to promote achievement rather than stressing punitive and pay-docking measures.
- *Include everyone.* Do not exclude hourly-paid employees. Remember that all employees perform some kind of service for someone. Their performance can be measured and they deserve the opportunity to excel and be recognized.
- *Reward teams, not just individuals.* Reinforce team play with team rewards, while also rewarding superior individual performers.

CHAPTER TWENTY-EIGHT

Make Your Office and Business More "Client Friendly"

You can't build a reputation on what you are going to do.

— Henry Ford

Another element of successful client and referral marketing is making your Home Care company more "client friendly."

Everybody likes doing business with friendly people. Your business is no exception.

Your Image Counts

Have a professional logo that carries throughout every aspect of communication with your clients — on uniforms, your stationery and business cards, invoices, newsletters, and other collateral material. You will be surprised at how much people do notice. The color of your business card, the type of brochure you produce, the copy in your ads — all of these can influence a buying decision. Most often potential clients are unable to *see* the difference between the quality of service your agency provides to that of your competition, so they look for agencies that represent professionalism and continuity!

Make sure your Home Care staff are well groomed, in clean uniforms, and wear nametags. Clients feel more comfortable when they know whom they are doing business with. Putting a name with a face makes people more accountable and approachable. It creates a friendly rapport.

Provide pictures of your office and supervisory staff to clients in "New Client Kits." Hang pictures of your staff on the wall of your business. This makes for a more human and friendly introduction to clients and prospective clients. It's nice to know what people look like who will be caring for you.

Make sure your offices are clean, warm, friendly, open, and approachable.

Educate and Include Your Staff

Provide employees with an opportunity to offer suggestions and ideas on how you can improve service delivery, reach prospective clients and referral sources. Ask for their help.

Provide an orientation for all employees regarding your image, your goals, and your marketing programs. You must get employees to support your efforts and become enthusiastic about working for a wonderful company.

Educate your employees on a regular basis. To make sure that your employees are handling calls correctly, have people call in to your office inquiring about services.

Give feedback to employees. You will appreciate and profit from these efforts.

- Your employees can be a wealth of referrals.
- An educated employee is much better equipped to answer a client's questions.
- Your employees will up-sell more often to clients as well as referral sources.

Handle Client Calls Courteously

Ensure that your telephones are answered promptly and that people are not placed on hold. *Training for all staff on telephone courtesy is critical.*

You should include a question or two on your client survey as to how they feel your staff have handled their telephone calls. Monitor this continuously.

Referral sources will also judge your service quality by the way in which their calls are handled. Since they may not have any other face-to-face interaction with your staff, the phone conversation may be their only basis to form judgments on how "people friendly" your business is and how you will treat other people.

Keep in Touch

Call clients, family members and referral sources often while your company is providing care to a person. Do not wait until there is a problem or until service is completed. Think about how you feel when your family doctor or dentist calls you after you have had an invasive procedure — just to see how you are doing. Home Care patients will appreciate having a call from the Nursing Supervisor to see how they are doing and if they are happy with the services. Obviously, face-to-face visits are more effective and should be used in addition to telephone calls.

Provide a constant flow of information to your clients. Send monthly newsletters, keeping clients informed and educated about your company. Send birthday or special occasion cards or a personal note when they are discharged. Keep in touch even after they are discharged. They may need your services again in the future. Plus they can be an excellent word-of-mouth referral source.

CHAPTER TWENTY-NINE

Review Services to Existing Clients

Rotate your vision every 1000 thoughts.

— Unknown

Home Care agencies can increase market share by attracting more new clients, providing more services for existing clients or referral sources, and reducing the loss of clients.

Formally marketing to existing clients addresses two out of the three. New client marketing is an intermediate step in the marketing process. What a company does *after* it converts a potential client to an actual client will go a long way toward determining that client's ultimate profitability.

Weekly Meetings

You must have a weekly meeting with your key staff in order to keep on track. The purpose of these meetings is to see how you are doing and to determine if you are meeting your goals.

Schedule an hour a week for this meeting and make it the same time every week. For instance: Tuesday from eight to nine A.M. — no exceptions. Do not change the schedule — pick the time and stick to it. Make sure that everyone knows this is a mandatory meeting.

Once a week! Not less often, not more often.

Here is an **action checklist** of questions that Home Care managers should ask concerning the effectiveness of the company's marketing to existing clients.

1. Do we know the profit impact of reducing our client defection rate by five percent? Have we communicated this information to all our staff, including hands-on caregivers as well as office staff and supervisors? Do they know the value of maintaining existent clients — for the company and themselves?

2. Do we plan our existing client marketing as carefully as we plan our new client marketing? Do we think in terms of creating true clients or just clients?

3. Do we stress value over price in our marketing? Do we feel that we have to buy our client loyalty?

4. Do we do all that we can to stay in touch with clients, resell the relationship, and say Thank You?

5. Do we encourage relationship-selling behaviors in our recruiting and training measures, and in how we compensate caregivers?
6. Do we focus enough energy on communication and customization?
7. Do we prize fairness in our company? Is fairness at the core of our company culture? When we make decisions that affect clients, do we make sure these decisions pass the fairness test?
8. Do we focus enough on competitive differentiation? Do we try to differentiate our whole company or do we rely mostly on one or two elements of the marketing mix to be distinctive.

CHAPTER THIRTY

Continually Review the Needs of the Market

Never leave well enough alone.

— Raymond Loewy

Smart marketing includes continually reviewing the changing needs and wants of clients and referral sources.

Assumptions about what clients want and feel often are wrong — because these can change! It is critical to continually perform market research, provide client questionnaires, and conduct focus groups.

Get Input from Employees

You must also listen to your front-line workers. The following questions should be provided to employees on a quarterly basis and employees should be provided an opportunity to respond confidentially to these questions:

- Would you refer a friend to work here?
- Would you have your parents or a family member cared for by this company?

- If you were President of this Home Care Company, what changes would you make to improve service, quality and morale?

Every quarter, the responses to these questionnaires should be shared with employees along with a plan to respond and improve any areas identified to be unsatisfactory. Also, suggestions for improvement should be shared with clients and referral sources in your monthly newsletter.

Get Input from Referral Sources

When conducting reviews, visit face-to-face with as many referral sources as possible. Make an appointment and *book for thirty minutes.* Explain that the purpose of your meeting is to re-evaluate your current service menu and that you respect their input and ideas. Ask them to *tell you* the ten most important features to be endorsed or recommended. Find out what they have not been happy about when dealing with other Home Care companies. Follow up with a sincere and detailed Thank You letter.

This is critical in building a trust bond with referral sources. Acknowledge their ideas and when you have implemented some or all of their recommendations you should let them know that you valued and acted on their ideas. Send these business contacts copies of your materials and a Thank You note crediting them for their help and ideas.

When employees, clients and referral sources actually see in writing how much emphasis you place on responding to suggestions, you will be amazed how positively they will respond. They will recognize that you really stand behind your commitment to quality.

CHAPTER THIRTY-ONE

Network Your Referral Sources

Never separate yourself from the community.
— Hillel

Why Clients Refer

1. **They trust that you will follow up** and make them feel good about making the referral.
2. **They think you are fair and competent.** People who refer Home Care clients require a sense of security and trust. They must feel that the patient will be well taken care of.
3. **You are convenient and easily accessible.** People today like things quick and easy. They want to be able to call one number, not be placed on hold, and be able to get immediate attention. If you can treat referrals as high priority, the response from referral sources will be very positive.
4. **Reciprocity is very important.** Setting up mutual referral systems is a quick, easy and professional way to generate more referrals.

Why People Don't Refer

1. **They think you are too busy** and that you will not be able to give their client the attention they need.

2. **They think you are too expensive.** Tell them your rates and explain why your rates are in the "highaverage" fee range. Stress the importance of attracting and retaining qualified home care staff and what services are included in your fees. Educate them. Although people say they look to low price first, psychologically they are afraid of it for fear that quality will be compromised.

3. **It never occurred to them to refer.** Plant the seeds in their mind that you welcome referrals and stress that you will not disappoint them or compromise their credibility by referring patients to you.

4. **They are afraid to be responsible for a referral** that would reflect poorly on their judgment. Work hard at increasing their confidence in you. Share testimonials or responses from existing client questionnaires.

5. **They have had a previous negative experience** with one of your competitors. Find out as much as possible from your potential referral sources what they did not like about other Home Care companies they have dealt with. You will have to convince potential referral sources why they should trust you and your staff, and why they should do business with you.

Marketing to Referral Sources

Do it right or don't do it!

Identify all of your current referral sources. Make a list of all potential referral sources in your community, including:

- Physicians
- Case Managers
- Social Workers
- Discharge Planners
- Directors of Care, Nursing Homes and Assisted Living Facilities
- Trust Officers
- Seniors Organizations
- Ministers
- Volunteer Organizations (i.e. Meals on Wheels)
- Local and State politicians
- Funeral Home Directors

Develop a strategic networking plan with input from your key management staff. Identify links or contacts with each of these referral groups.

Identify all community and state associations and determine the value of attending meetings and workshops. Develop a plan of who should represent your company at these meetings.

Position your company as a resource to the community when it comes to Home Care services. Provide information not only about your services but also about industry statistics, regulations, new trends, etc. Develop a package of information that you can provide to these contacts. Send copies of newsletters, press releases, brochures or industry information on a regular basis. This will set you apart from other companies.

This is the essence of effective networking — *helping others.* This is one of the fastest ways to cultivate productive relationships. When you help others you will get much more in return.

Be sure your staff members know that client referral sources are essential to the future of your business, so they will give them proper recognition and attention. Give acknowledgment in newsletters and memos to employees who refer clients to your agency.

Six Ways to Encourage Clients, Staff and Friends to Refer

1. **Ask them!**
   Develop your own technique, with which you feel most comfortable.

2. **Reward referrals.**
   Thank employees with a dinner-for-two, flowers, fruit baskets, etc. Send thank you letters, or call referral sources and thank them for trusting your company. Try to send an unusual card, that will be saved or displayed, with your name, logo, address, and phone number in full view. Or give them a magnet or coffee mug with your logo. They will look at it every day.

3. **Keep in touch with referral sources.**
   Let them know how the person whom they referred to you is progressing under your care.

4. **Refer business to them.**
   Everyone likes to feel that he or she is getting what he or she wants or needs. For example: if you are getting referrals from an Assisted Living Facility, ask if you could

have your nursing staff visit the facility for the purpose of orientating your staff. Often facilities will rely on Home Care staff to refer or endorse Nursing Homes or Assisted Living Facilities.

5. **Believe in your quality and service level.**
   If you don't commit to quality, why should anyone refer you?

6. **Seek out referrals from competitors.**
   Some of your best referrals can come from your apparent "competitors." For example: other Home Care companies may not be able to fill the shifts or service a particular geographic area. If you can set up reciprocal referring relationships, you may be surprised how much this can help your business.

CHAPTER THIRTY-TWO

Track Referrals

Dig your well before you're thirsty.

— Harvey Mackay

You should absolutely track every referral your Home Care agency receives. Without implementing a system to track referrals, you will not be able to evaluate the effectiveness of your marketing efforts and, more importantly, you will not be able to acknowledge and thank your referral sources.

A simple-to-use referral form is provided for you to use — or you can design your own.

- Orient every person in your agency on how to complete this form when they take a new referral — whether they are answering a call during regular hours, after hours or on weekends. Commitment from everyone is key.
- Once a week, appoint someone in each office to summarize a list of referrals received and the source of each referral.
- Use the list to generate your thank you letters and acknowledgments in your newsletters. Circulate the list to all your staff weekly if possible and at least monthly.

- Use your collected statistics of referral patterns to monitor the effectiveness of your staff's face-to-face meetings with referral sources, trade and health fairs and marketing programs.

You will be amazed after tracking referrals to learn that 80% of your referrals are being generated from 20% of your contacts.

Intake/Referral Form

Patient: ______________________ Date of Birth: __________ Age: __________

Address: ______________________ Medicare # : ______________________

City, State: ______________________ Medicaid # : ______________________

Zip Code: __________ Telephone: __________ Social Security # : ______________________

Physician: ______________________ Private Insurance Co.: ______________________

Address: ______________________ Group#: __________ Policy #: __________

Telephone: ______________________ Hospital or SNF: ______________________

Responsible Party: ______________________ Admission: __________ Discharge: __________

Address: ______________________ Previous Agency Patient?: ______________________

Telephone: ______________________ Referred By: ______________________

Diagnosis Primary: ______________________

Secondary: ______________________

Disciplines:

	Check	Frequency of Visits
R.N.		
H.H.A.		
P.T.		
S.T.		
O.T.		
M.S.W.		
Hmkr.		
Live-In		

Medications/Treatment ______________________

Physician's Orders: ______________________

Level of Staff Requested ______________________

Diet: ______________________ Allergies: ______________________

Precautions: ______________________

Comments: ______________________

Person taking referral: ______________________ Date: __________

Referral given to: ______________________ Date: __________

M.D. verbal orders given by: ______________________ Date: __________

Signature: ______________________ Date: __________

75% OF ORIGINAL SIZE

CHAPTER THIRTY-THREE

Courtesy and Appreciation for Clients

Thank you, thank you very much.
— Elvis Presley

Every person who works in the Home Care Industry should understand why and how clients are lost. Obviously, clients are lost if they had a temporary condition and they have improved. Sometimes clients no longer qualify for Medicare coverage, or a client's financial situation may change. But, other than these scenarios, are you aware of the main reasons clients no longer use a Home Care agency's services?

- 68% of lost clients are the direct result of staff discourtesy.
- 16% are lost due to service dissatisfaction.
- 11% are lost to competitive inroads.
- 4% simply move (may go into institution).
- 1% pass away
  (see diagram on next page)

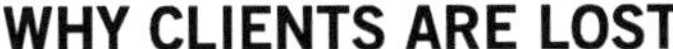

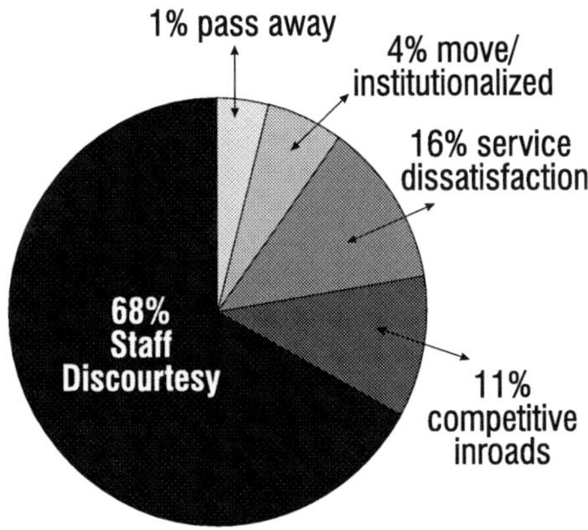

Courtesy counts.

When the lack of basic courtesy and client appreciation affects your business *this much*, education about courtesy must become part of your "marketing plan."

- All of your personnel must be courteous, even when difficult situations present themselves. Teach your staff how to handle difficult clients and difficult circumstances.
- Ask questions to establish trust and to ensure that you are able to determine what is important to the other party. Present solutions to that party, which are specifically tailored to meet their needs.
- Give clients your full attention. Your staff must make each client or referral source feel — at that moment — that they are the most important person in the world.
- Communicate often with your clients, both in writing and in person. You should continually be looking for ways to ensure your clients are happy with your service and your staff.

- Be convinced your clients need the services you are offering and focus on the benefits your client receives as a result of using your services.

Note: Most people will not complain. They will find excuses to cancel services if they are unhappy. Unless you have established a method to constantly monitor and get feedback from the client, you will be unable to predict and actively attend to potential dissatisfaction.

Plan for Client Appreciation

- Make it your agency's commitment to continually show appreciation to your clients.
- Send thank you cards or letters and write personal notes.
- Make sure you have your client's birthdays and anniversaries on file and send flowers.

We struck up a relationship with a local florist and provided them our coffee mugs with the company's logo. We negotiated a discounted price for special floral mug arrangements to be delivered to our clients. We were able to provide the florist with a guaranteed number of arrangements per month and this enabled us to get a very good deal.

We assigned one person in each office to provide the florist with the names and addresses every month of our appreciation list — and we didn't have to worry about anything. The florist took care of it for us. This worked very well for us — plus the clients and their families loved it! For Christmas we gave tins of cookies with our name on them to our special clients.

I love newsletters because they also provide an opportunity to recognize clients' special birthdays and anniversaries. Newsletters are a very easy, inexpensive way to keep in constant contact with your clients. Even after you discharge a client, keep them on your mailing list for newsletters. Think of it this way — for every month you don't contact your clients, that client loses ten percent of the value of your relationship.

If a client feels ignored — even though she is receiving adequate care — she may look elsewhere for service. Very rarely can a client be lured away to another agency if she feels appreciated and loved by her current Home Care agency.

CHAPTER THIRTY-FOUR

Respond to Complaints — *Fast*

Everything you do or say is public relations.

— Unknown

Always respond to complaints quickly and efficiently.

Never leave a client or referral source unhappy — even if it is a difficult client and you want to get rid of them.

If you give a client their money back, they can't say bad things about you. If you don't, they'll go to all ends to tell everyone they know what a terrible company you are.

Use a form complaint response letter but make sure you personalize it. (See Complaint Response Letter in Chapter 46.)

Keep in mind the Lifetime Value of a Client (LVC). The LVC is the total profit produced by an average client over their lifetime association with you. (This is usually considered to be one year.) Start calculating the lifetime value of your average client. By doing this calculation and sharing this information with your staff, you will begin to look at your clients in a much different light.

CHAPTER THIRTY-FIVE

The Power of the Phone

The difference between ordinary and extraordinary is that little extra.
— Unknown

Many businesses treat the inbound call as an interruption to work rather than "opportunity calling." Advertising campaigns can only be evaluated as being successful when they generate calls. Why then do we not invest as much time and money on preparing our staff for these calls?

Smart businesses invest the time and money in training their staff on telephone etiquette as well as telephone sales.

Expecting a receptionist with no training or incentives — and often with competing and conflicting responsibilities — to do a great job "selling" to inbound callers is a drastic mistake. The position of receptionist must not be underrated nor undervalued. This is often the first voice a potential client hears. What will it say about your company?

Each impression you make may be your last.

If a prospective client calls your office inquiring about Home Care services, remember they may never have heard about your company before seeing your ad or brochure. If they call your office and they are fortunate enough to speak to someone who is enthusiastic, informative, caring, and who provides useful information, it is highly likely your company will end up on the top of the list.

Call around to other Home Care companies inquiring about their services. Find out how friendly your *competitors* are on the phone.

Voice Mail

Many people do not like voice mail and they resent being placed on hold, forced into listening to annoying or inappropriate music.

Consider investing the money in a voice *message* system. That way when anyone is placed on hold, they can hear about your company history and the services you provide. Including real testimonials from clients as part of your taped message can also be powerful.

Do not waste this precious opportunity to let clients — and other callers who may be potential clients — learn more about your business.

CHAPTER THIRTY-SIX

New Client Kit

Your true value depends entirely on what you are compared with.

— Bob Wells

The selection of a Home Care agency is a confusing decision for a client. Many people lack familiarity with the health care system to make wellinformed decisions. When they are in need of service, it usually follows a medical crisis and this can be a very difficult time to make a well-informed decision.

Clients are likely to have tremendous fear and anxiety related to the unknown and questions regarding the economic consequences. Providers must be very generous with information that can assist the client and family — not only in making the right decision, but also in managing expectations.

- It is extremely important not to raise expectations you cannot meet.
- Client satisfaction is the gap between what the client expects and what is received.
- To manage satisfaction you must carefully manage your client's satisfaction.

This is why a "New Client Kit" is absolutely critical.

What should a "New Client Kit" contain?

- Thank-you Letter from the owner/CEO
- Information about your Agency and its Services
- Emergency Procedures
- List of Testimonials from other clients
- New Client Questionnaire
- Company Policies
- Clinical Information
- Client Care Plan
- Photographs of Care-givers
- An issue of your Newsletter
- Copy of Signed Consent
- New Client Checklist that has been signed by the supervisor acknowledging that everything has been explained and understood by the client.

NEW CLIENT KIT EXAMPLE

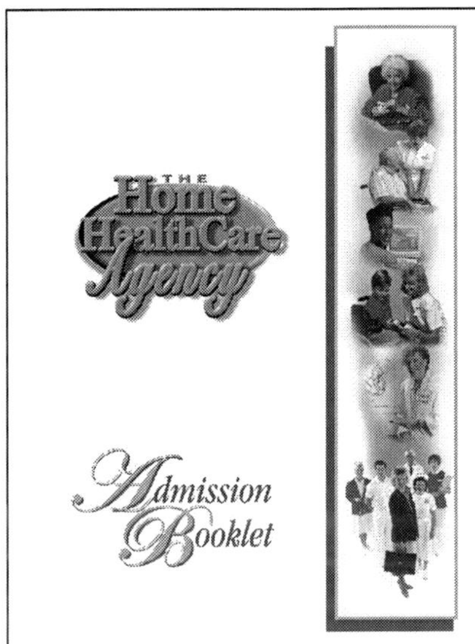

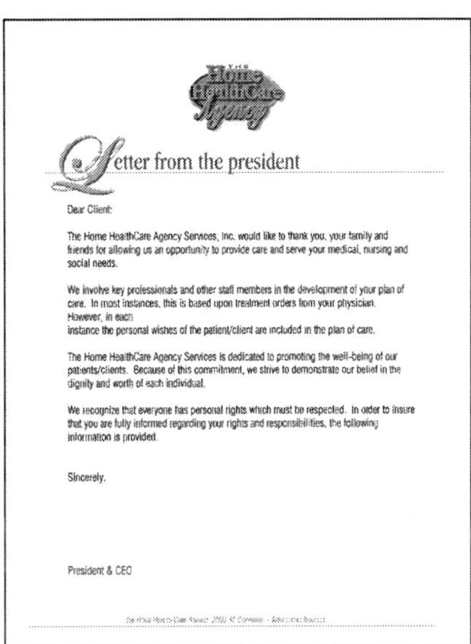

Letter from the president

Dear Client:

The Home HealthCare Agency Services, Inc. would like to thank you, your family and friends for allowing us an opportunity to provide care and serve your medical, nursing and social needs.

We involve key professionals and other staff members in the development of your plan of care. In most instances, this is based upon treatment orders from your physician. However, in each
instance the personal wishes of the patient/client are included in the plan of care.

The Home HealthCare Agency Services is dedicated to promoting the well-being of our patients/clients. Because of this commitment, we strive to demonstrate our belief in the dignity and worth of each individual.

We recognize that everyone has personal rights which must be respected. In order to insure that you are fully informed regarding your rights and responsibilities, the following information is provided.

Sincerely,

President & CEO

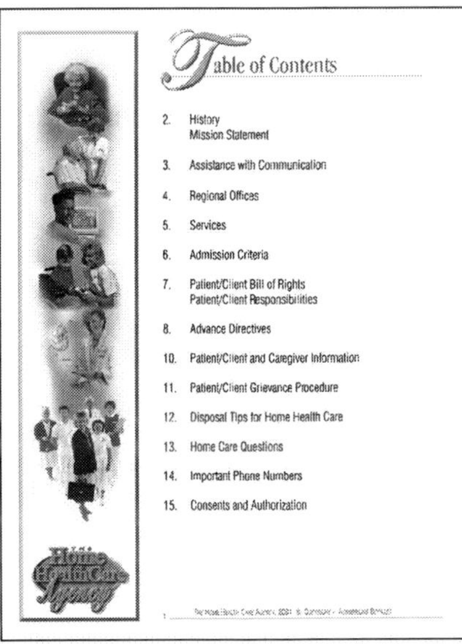

Table of Contents

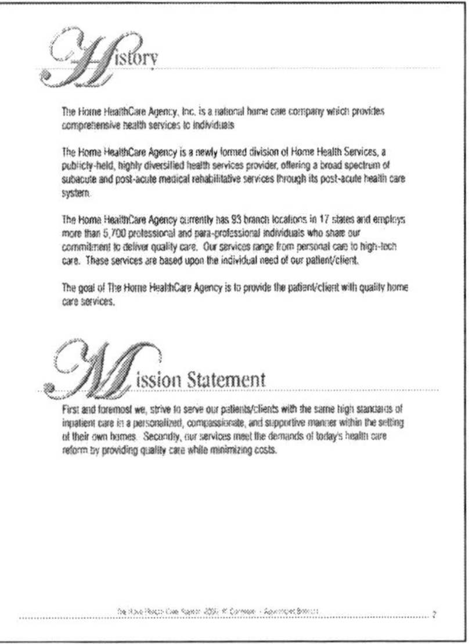

History

The Home HealthCare Agency, Inc. is a national home care company which provides comprehensive health services to individuals

The Home HealthCare Agency is a newly formed division of Home Health Services, a publicly-held, highly diversified health services provider, offering a broad spectrum of subacute and post-acute medical rehabilitative services through its post-acute health care system.

The Home HealthCare Agency currently has 93 branch locations in 17 states and employs more than 5,700 professional and para-professional individuals who share our commitment to deliver quality care. Our services range from personal care to high-tech care. These services are based upon the individual need of our patient/client.

The goal of The Home HealthCare Agency is to provide the patient/client with quality home care services.

Mission Statement

First and foremost we, strive to serve our patients/clients with the same high standards of inpatient care in a personalized, compassionate, and supportive manner within the setting of their own homes. Secondly, our services meet the demands of today's health care reform by providing quality care while minimizing costs.

NEW CLIENT KIT EXAMPLE CONTINUED

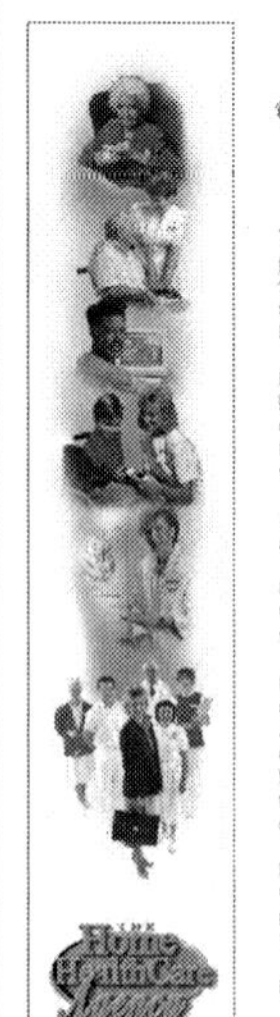

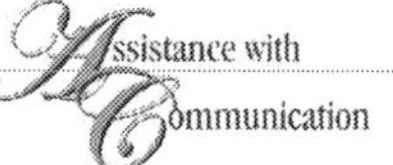

The Home HealthCare Agency recognizes that many patients/clients face communication challenges due to hearing, speech or visual impairment. In addition, we recognize that some individuals communicate in a language other than English

In some cases, The Home HealthCare Agency personnel may be able to communicate with patients/clients in a language other than English. When this is not the case, The Home HealthCare Agency has made arrangements with_________________to provide interpreter services

(For those who experience either hearing or speech difficulties, an interpreter will be available).

If you require or desire having this service, or if our staff think it would be helpful to have an interpreter assist you, arrangements will be made to use this service at no additional cost to you.

If it is determined that a language interpreter will be used in meeting your needs, arrangements will be made to have such an individual assist us in any in-person or telephone communication with you. The interpreter will be contacted by telephone and help us communicate by translating information for you and a member of the The Home HealthCare Agency staff.

For those who have hearing or speech difficulties, arrangements will be made to use a TTY/TDD service. The hearing impaired number is
1-800-000-0000

If you have visual difficulties, arrangements will be made to

3

Regional Offices

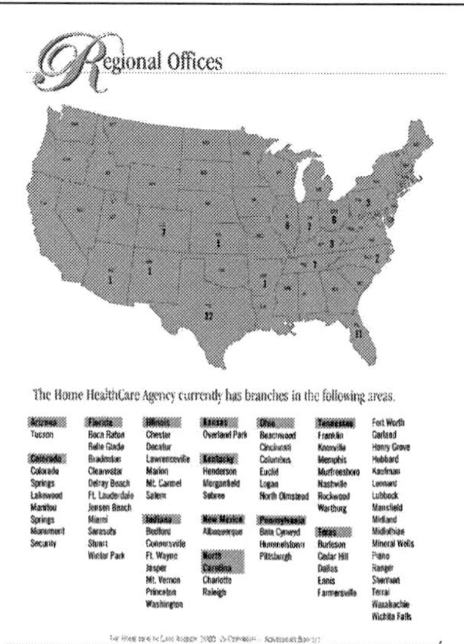

The Home HealthCare Agency currently has branches in the following areas.

Arizona
Tucson

Colorado
Colorado Springs
Lakewood
Manitou Springs
Monument
Security

Florida
Boca Raton
Belle Glade
Bradenton
Clearwater
Delray Beach
Ft. Lauderdale
Jensen Beach
Miami
Sarasota
Stuart
Winter Park

Illinois
Chester
Decatur
Lawrenceville
Marion
Mt. Carmel
Salem

Indiana
Bedford
Connersville
Ft. Wayne
Jasper
Mt. Vernon
Princeton
Washington

Kansas
Overland Park

Kentucky
Henderson
Morganfield
Sebree

New Mexico
Albuquerque

North Carolina
Charlotte
Raleigh

Ohio
Beachwood
Cincinnati
Columbus
Euclid
Logan
North Olmstead

Pennsylvania
Bala Cynwyd
Hummelstown
Pittsburgh

Tennessee
Franklin
Knoxville
Memphis
Murfreesboro
Nashville
Rockwood
Wartburg

Texas
Burleson
Cedar Hill
Dallas
Ennis
Farmersville
Fort Worth
Garland
Honey Grove
Hubbard
Kaufman
Leonard
Lubbock
Mansfield
Midland
Midlothian
Mineral Wells
Plano
Ranger
Sherman
Terrell
Waxahachie
Wichita Falls

4

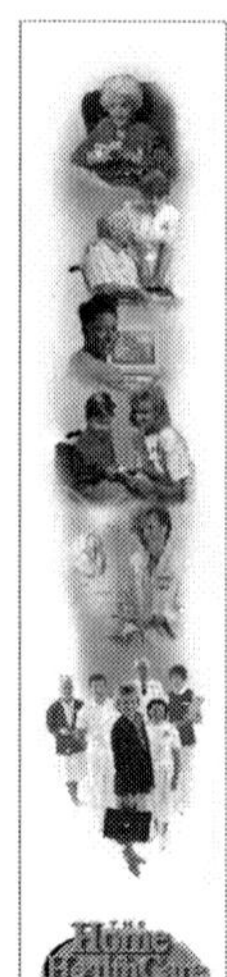

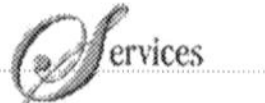

Making a difference in people's lives.

- Skilled Nursing
- Medical Social Worker
- Speech Pathology
- Occupational Therapy
- Physical Therapy
- Home Health Aide
- Homemakers

Speciality Services

- Maternal Infant Care Services
- Oncology Services
- Pediatric Services
- Psychiatric Services
- Respiratory Services
- Enterostomal Therapy
- Infusion Therapy
- Diabetic Management
- Home Medical Equipment

Some services may not be available in certain locations. In some instances, The Home HealthCare Agency may furnish one of the services listed above through a contractual relationship with another company. Patients/Clients will be notified when services are provided by other companies under contract with The Home HealthCare Agency.

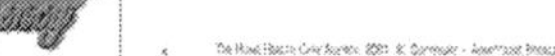

5

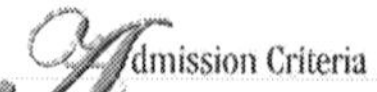

Admission to this agency is based on patient/client needs, homebound status and the type of services required which can be provided by this company. In order to make a determination about suitability for home care, it is important to provide relevant information during the admissions process thus, your cooperation is imperative. We encourage you to permit members of your family and those assisting you in your home to share relevant information with us in order to complete a comprehensive admission process.

Policies: This book contains general information regarding your rights and responsibilities as a patient/client. As state and federal regulations change, there may be additions or alterations to this book as necessary. The complete policy and procedure manual regarding your care and treatment is available upon request for your viewing at any time during normal business hours.

Ownership: This agency is owned by The Home HealthCare Agency, Inc/IHS, and in compliance with: Title VI of the Civil Rights Act of 1964; section 504 of the Rehabilitation Act of 1973; the Americans with Disabilities Act; and the Age Discrimination Act of 1975. The Home HealthCare Agency does not discriminate on the basis of race, creed, color, age, gender, national origin, or disability in admission ,access to treatment or employment. The administration will coordinate all efforts to comply with these laws and relevant regulatory requirements.

Payment: Reimbursement for services may be provided through Medicare, Medicaid, Worker's Compensation, Veterans Administration Insurance, Private Insurance, Managed Care Organization, Private Pay, or Credit Card. For some services, there is no charge to the patient/client if they are eligible for Medicare or Medicaid. Any charges for services not covered under Titles XVII and XIX of the Social Security Act or nonreimbursable charges will be discussed with you prior to rendering these services. Prior to, or on admission, the patient/client, guardian, caregiver or family member will be informed of all charges for services to be provided and method of payment. Should any change be made in this policy regarding services or charges, you or your responsible party will be advised.

Patient/Client needs: Our policy is to admit only those individuals for whom we can reasonably meet demonstrated needs in care and service. On an ongoing basis, we monitor patient/client needs. When situations occur in which patient/client needs can no longer be accommodated, either by The Home HealthCare Agency personnel or through service provided by other agencies, we will develop a discharge or transfer plan for the individual.

Safety and Security: The safety and security of patients/clients and our personnel are key considerations. As such, in those instances in which safety and security are in jeopardy, we reserve the right to withdraw service without prior notification to either the patient/client or referral source.

6

NEW CLIENT KIT EXAMPLE CONTINUED

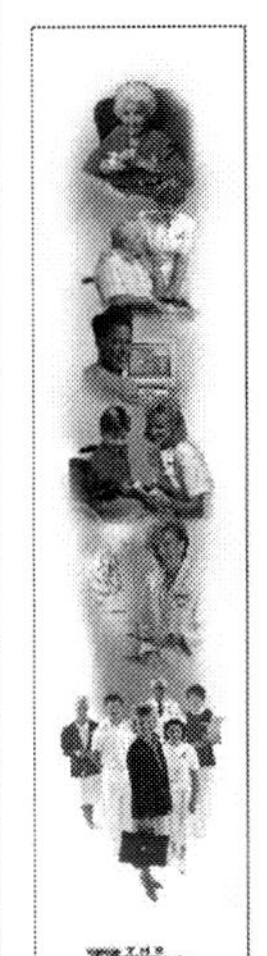

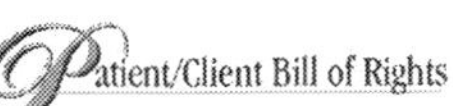

Patient/Client Bill of Rights

The Home HealthCare Agency recognizes that the patient/client has the right:

- To competent, professional individualized care without regard to race, creed, color, age, gender, physical handicap or national origin.
- To have his/her privacy respected and to know all case related information will be kept confidential to the extent permitted by law.
- To a written plan of care designed to meet individual needs.
- To know the names and titles of those individuals responsible for coordinating, rendering or supervising his/her care.
- To participate in all decisions regarding the plan of treatment and to refuse any procedure or treatment.
- To examine, question, and receive a full explanation of any invoice and to review the record of his/her care at any time.
- To be fully informed of the policies of The Home HealthCare Agency and the charges of care.
- To receive care from qualified personnel who are experienced in the skills and procedures necessary at levels of understanding in their respective field of employment.
- To expect recommended services, evaluations and referrals appropriate to the nature of his/her diagnosis and rehabilitation plan.
- To contact a designated The Home HealthCare Agency supervisor 24 hours per day, 7 days a week.
- To report abusive, neglectful or exploitative practices of health care workers or the agency.

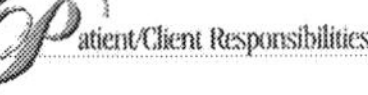

Patient/Client Responsibilities

The Home HealthCare Agency also recognizes that the patient/client has certain responsibilities. These include the following:

- To carry out the plan of care, as instructed, to arrive at the highest level of health and level of wellness and independence as can be achieved in the content of the patient's/client's condition.
- To treat agency personnel with courtesy, respect and without regard, to race, creed, color, age, gender, physical handicap or national origin.

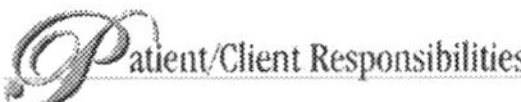

Patient/Client Responsibilities

- To provide the agency with current, accurate information regarding health care needs and reimbursement information essential to the provision of services.
- To participate to the extent possible in decisions regarding the development, implementation, and revision of the plan of care.
- To inform the agency on a timely basis of any dissatisfaction or questions about agency services.
- To furnish a written authorization for release of information essential for the provision of quality care reimbursement.
- To make prompt payment for agency services in accordance with his/her financial responsibility or to inform the agency on a timely basis of any difficulty in making payments and to request a satisfactory payment schedule.

It is understood and agreed that in those instances in which family members participate in the care, assistance or supervision of the patient/client, they share the responsibilities described above.

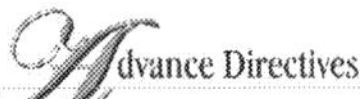

Advance Directives

An Advance Directive is a written instruction that expresses an individual's wishes regarding health care to be furnished to the individual when he or she is unable to make a treatment decision. The intent of the advance directive is to enhance the individual's control over medical treatment decisions.

Depending upon the state in which you reside, an advance directive can take many forms. This includes a living will, a durable power of attorney for health care, or a health care proxy.

Some definitions help clarify the nature and purpose of advance directives:

A Living Will is a document that describes the types of treatment that the individual wishes to receive after he or she can no longer make health care choices. Most living wills only become effective when the person is terminally ill.

A Durable Power of Attorney in Health Care designates a person to serve as the decision-maker for health care choices for patient/client when he or she is unable to do so. Many individuals also furnish the designated person with a set of requests or instructions to help make treatment choices.

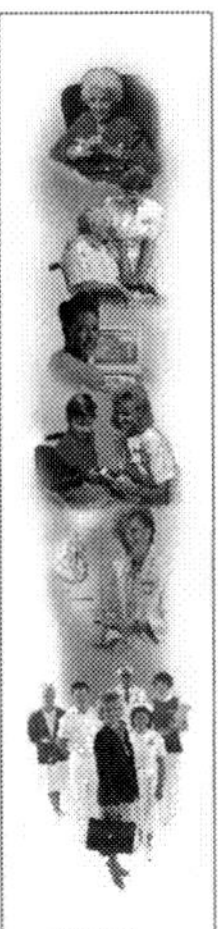

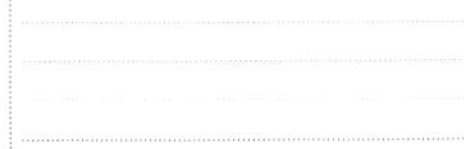

Advance Directives

A Health Care Proxy fulfills much the same role as a durable power of attorney in health care. This is designated according to state laws.

Do Not Resuscitate requests are addressed in some advance directives as the patient/client requests the right to refuse resuscitation.

"Do Not Hospitalize" or "Do Not Transport". Some states have passed laws that recognize the right of a home care patient/client to refuse to be transported to a hospital or other urgent care treatment facility. Many hospice and severely ill home care patients/clients make such requests.

You are not required to complete an advance directive. However, if you choose to do so, The Home HealthCare Agency will maintain a copy of your advance directive in your clinical record and our staff will be informed. In this way we can assist in honoring the requests made in your advance directive.

Each state has different requirements regarding advance directives. You will find in the admission packet details about advance directives in accordance with the laws of your jurisdiction. The Home HealthCare Agency will honor it to the extent permitted by local law.

The Home HealthCare Agency will inform the patient/client, staff, and community of up-dated information as it relates to the advance directives.

Patients/Clients who have a advance directive and wish to voice concern about the implementation of the advance directive may call the Toll-free Home Health Agency hot line phone number.____________________
The hot line is in operation between___AM through___PM____
____days per week.

Additional State or Local Information:

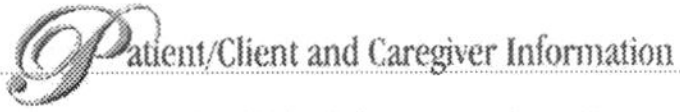

Patient/Client and Caregiver Information

We encourage your input: The goal of The Home HealthCare Agency is to provide patients/clients with quality home care services. To assist us in meeting this goal, we encourage you to call our office to voice your suggestions for improving our services. Our office hours are from ___AM to ___PM Monday through Friday. Please feel free to phone us with your suggestions by dialing__________________ and ask to speak with________________________.

In addition, we want you to know that you may be asked to participate in customer satisfaction surveys that are designed to assist us in improving our home care programs. Patients/Clients are chosen at random for this purpose. You do not have to take part in these surveys; however, we value your input in our effort to continuously improve our home care service. Therefore, we encourage your participation in our patient/client satisfaction surveys.

How to Work Effectively with Home Care Personnel: Having home care staff work with you or a family member may be a new experience. Home care staff are trained to provide care or service in a manner that is as least disruptive as the situation permits. Our staff will look to you to orient them to your home. Please feel free to share with our staff information that may impact your care.

Although efforts will be made to assign the same staff to assist you during each visit, this may not always be possible to achieve. The Home HealthCare Agency reserves the right to substitute staff. In addition, just as we respect your cultural and religious beliefs, we have the same regard for the beliefs of our staff. Therefore, we may substitute personnel in those situations in which the services required conflict with the individual's philosophical or religious beliefs.

We ask all our patients/clients to refrain from asking our staff to perform services beyond the scope of the plan of care. Repeated requests may result in a decision to terminate service. Similarly, any evidence of abuse, harassment, or threatened assault will result in prompt discontinuance of service.

How to be an effective Caregiver for the Patient/Client: During the admissions process, a member of the Home HealthCare Agency staff will discuss a number of matters with you, including the plan of care, diagnosis, medications, diet, and staffing requirements. A checklist is included in this admissions booklet that will serve as a reminder for you that these matters were discussed.

Between visits by The Home HealthCare Agency staff, you may notice changes in the patient's/client's condition that are of concern to you. DO NOT WAIT until the next visit to report these conditions to the staff.

CONTACT your case manager_______________________________, or in URGENT CASES, CALL 911.

It is always appreciated if you notify our staff when safety becomes an issue, including when furniture has been rearranged or when equipment used in providing service is in disrepair. In this way, appropriate steps can be taken to correct potential safety concerns.

We are also including in this section some tips for those caregivers who must dispose of sharp objects, soiled bandages, sheets, and medical gloves. Our staff will review this information with you.

Enclosed, you will find a handy insert of Important Telephone Numbers. We encourage you to complete it and place it near your telephone. It is a useful reference for important calls that you may need to make to the doctor, pharmacist, or other family members.

CHAPTER THIRTY-SEVEN

Add More Services

Try new things. Encourage your staff and the agency to look for the great idea. When it comes, the heavens open.

— Leo Greenland

You should constantly evaluate your "service menu" and determine whether there are other services your company could be offering to complement your service mix.

It's very easy to sit still and wait for your competitors to come up with new ideas and then try to replicate their services. But remember the *Law of Leadership: It is better to be first than it is to be better.* One reason the first brand tends to maintain its leadership is that the name often becomes well known and generic.

When you launch a new service, the first question to ask yourself is *not* "How is this new service better than what is offered by my competitors?" but "What new category is this service in?" Everyone is interested in what is *new.*

A company can become incredibly successful if it can find a way to brand a new service — to "own" a word or phase in the mind of the prospect.

"Shared Care"

This is an example of one service we launched in the market that was very successful because the term "Shared Care" became associated with our company.

Here is how it happened.

Our company had developed an excellent relationship in one of our markets with an Assisted Living Facility.

When we opened our office we had called on the administration of the Assisted Living Facility and met to discuss the potential of providing private duty services to any of their residents when they required more assistance than the facility staff could provide.

The occupancy rate of the Assisted Living Facility was less than fifty percent and the administrator was struggling in trying to fill up the rooms.

During the next several months, we worked closely to try to come up with ways we could cross-market our services.

We identified that some of the Assisted Living Facility's existing clients did require a few hours a day of assistance. We designed a program where we assigned one home care aide to work with two clients on the same floor. We developed a care plan for each client and assigned specific tasks and time schedules for the home care aide to follow. Instead of charging our regular hourly rate, we came up with a reduced hourly rate, which saved money for the client *and* enabled us to give our home care aide a premium hourly rate for caring for two patients.

The clients loved it and the employees loved it — because they didn't have to travel between clients and they made more money.

The Assisted Living Facility used this co-servicing relationship as a selling advantage. The availability of "Shared Care" boosted the benefits of their facility and their marketing stance. Within the next several months the Assisted Living Facility filled and our caseload grew to a point that we had three or four home care aides working full time.

We packaged this new service, "Shared Care," developed brochures and other collateral material, and began to market to other Assisted Living Facilities in other cities (see example on next page).

This new service became the foundation of our company's services to Assisted Living Facilities and was very profitable. Over time we expanded into supplemental staffing to these facilities, and private duty services for residents who required short-term acute care.

Our company was the first Home Care company in our market to offer this type of service — and the term "Shared Care" then became a generic term used by our competitors. Because we were *first* in using and creating it, we were recognized for having pioneered this program.

SHARED CARE BROCHURE SAMPLE

Call Our Office
Today
For Further Information
THE Home HealthCare Agency
123 Anystreet
Anytown, USA
12334
1-800-555-1234
When You Only
Need A Little Help
Shared Care

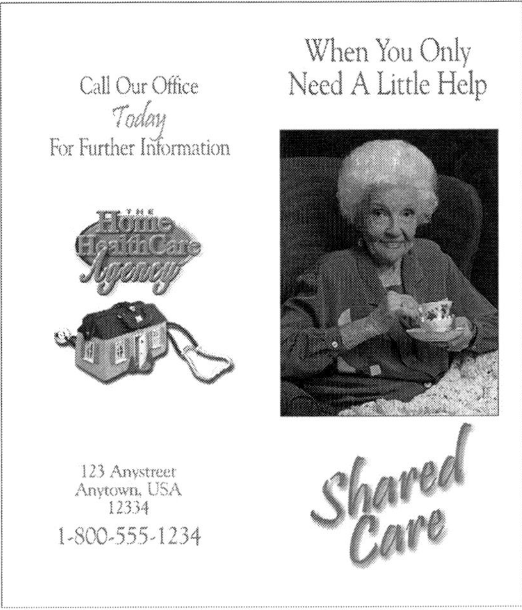

OUTSIDE: 35% OF ORIGINAL SIZE

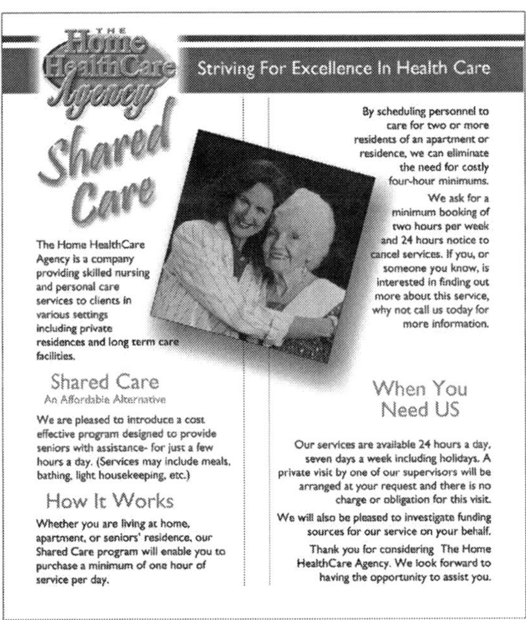

INSIDE: 35% OF ORIGINAL SIZE

CHAPTER THIRTY-EIGHT

Package and Up-Sell Your Services to Existing Clients

The most important order you get from a customer is the second order. Why? Because a two-time buyer is at least twice as likely to buy again as a one-time buyer.

— Bob Stone

Do not forget that your existing and former clients are your best sources of new business revenue.

If a client has been receiving skilled services covered by Medicare or insurance, you should, prior to discharging that client, determine whether he or she could benefit from custodial care or assistance with personal care. Even though they may not qualify for Medicare-covered care, they may be willing to pay privately for services.

Keeping in touch with former clients by phone and mail *after* discharge will ensure that, if they should require assistance, you will be in a position to respond quickly.

Our experience from maintaining regular calls and calling existing clients prior to discharge was very positive. Over 44% of our clients were topping up their government-funded or insurance-covered care with out-of-pocket private services.

You have to go after this business — clients generally don't bring it up. Unless clients know that they can purchase services privately and that they can keep the same homemaker or attendant, you may never get the business.

You should be able to up-sell 20% of your clients. Up-selling means selling additional services and/or products to existing clients.

If you could up-sell 20% of your clients on six hours of homemaking services per week, calculate the potential profit. Here is an example:

If you currently serve 500 clients, a 20% up-sell equals 100 of those clients. 100 clients at $14.00 an hour times 52 weeks is equal to $436,800 in increased sales for the year. If you are running a 10% profit margin, *this comes out to $43,680 additional profits per year.*

Create packages of services for your clients vs. Cafeteria Selling

I encourage you to bundle your services into packages and stay away from "cafeteria" selling. By packaging your services you will *increase your average sale amount.* In additon you will:

- Increase value of each client
- Increase value to your clients
- Be able to plan in advance for staff selection

- Keep clients *connected* to you
- MD's and referral sources will benefit from ongoing communication regarding the client's progress.

Examples of Care Packages

Plan #1 $300.00/month

- One RN/LVN visit per month
- 6 hours per week of Homemaking services
- Telephone check once/week
- 24 hour call-in

Plan #2 $200.00/month

- One RN/LVN visit every 60 days
- 3 hours per week of Homemaking services
- Call from nurse once per week

Here are some other services to consider packaging

- Medication reminder calls
- Morning and evening personal care visits
- Housecleaning services
- Companion care

Another service to offer is case-management. A case-manager provides follow-ups, makes sure the client gets to medical appointments, checks on medical status and keeps out-of-town family informed on the progress of their loved one.

Send out questionnaires monthly to existing clients, former clients, referral sources, and family members of clients asking for suggestions of other services they are interested in — *and follow up.*

CHAPTER THIRTY-NINE

Special Offers — the Cash Surge

There comes a moment when you have to stop revving up the car and shove it into gear.

— David Mahoney

If your business revenue has been declining, consider implementing a "cash flow surge program" by sending a letter to former clients and referral sources offering a discount to be applied against their invoice.

Obviously, this will only be attractive to clients who are in need of inhome support and who may be deciding on whether to purchase home care services. Referral sources can provide a "discount coupon" to patients who are in need of care — and, in the process, feel good about giving their clients something.

You may not think this is appropriate for Home Care marketing, but seniors love discounts and appreciate it when you offer them a chance to save money.

When you offer a savings opportunity, have a good reason. Here are examples of a few "good reasons."

> "We are offering this value only to our former clients as a reward for their support."
>
> "We're extending this offering only to new, first-time clients."
>
> "We have an experienced Home Care team eager to work with you and thought that offering this exceptional value would be a good reason for you to call us."

Offer a coupon or gift certificate.

Lots of people like to give friends and family members gift certificates for services such as spa days, massages, etc. Consider having a gift certificate printed — offering a 5–10% discount on first billing for hourly care. Include the certificate in your newsletters, direct mail and even your web site.

THE Home HealthCare Agency

Call 24 hours a day, 7 days a week!

GIFT CERTIFICATE

10% Discount on First Billing.

Phone: (555) 555-5555
Toll Free: (800) 555-5555
Fax: (555) 555-5554

Name: ______________________________

Address: ______________________________

City: ________________ State: __________ Zip: __________

Phone: ______________________________

Email: ______________________________

CHAPTER FORTY

Become a Source of Information

The secret of success is to know something nobody else knows.

— Aristotle Onassis

Keeping your clients educated about your company, the health care industry, their medical condition and related treatments should be an integral part of your service package. Know as much as possible about diseases, ailments, conditions, treatments and services options. You can build tremendous loyalty by making sure your clients are provided information about their treatment or illness.

Clients want to know about your company, but they also really want to know about the industry in general. If you are positioned as an agency that educates, you will attract more business and earn more trust.

Consider developing a checklist for people to use when seeking a Home Care provider. (See example) You can use this checklist to position your company and set yourself apart from your competitors.

Check List for Selecting a Home Care Provider

Ask for recommendations from Physicians, Hospital Case Managers.
Call various home care companies and ask the following questions:

Agency Name:____

	Yes	No
1. Is your agency Medicare certified?	☐	☐
2. Are your staff insured, bonded?	☐	☐
3. Are your services available 7 days/week?	☐	☐
4. How are your staff supervised?	☐	☐
5. Will your supervisor make a home visit prior to services commencing?	☐	☐
6. How do you select your caregivers____________________		
7. How do you train your employees? ____________________		
8. Can I meet your staff in advance?	☐	☐
9. What happens if your caregiver is sick?____________________		
10. What are your rates? And minimum hours of service? ____________		
11. When do you send out invoices? ____________________		
12. What services does your agency offer?____________________		
13. What duties will your staff not perform?____________________		
14. Can your agency provide references?	☐	☐

Make Use of All Materials

Using your website, newsletters, letters and client-directed education manuals, you will set yourself apart from your competitors.

Your Website

I believe that you can also use your website effectively to educate clients as well as employees. Through a website, you can establish your company as being a leader and provider of information.

Do not underestimate how effective a website can be in positioning your company. In many cases it is a daughter or family member who is charged with finding home care service for a parent or relative. That person will appreciate the accessibility of information — not only about you but also about health care issues in general. Referral sources such as case managers, social workers and physicians can also access your site. Many potential clients or referral sources will use your site as a way to perform initial research about your company, and then call your number to get more specific information.

Handbooks and Manuals

Handbooks and training manuals are also very powerful tools. We developed a pediatric guidebook for parents, describing various procedures to assist families and caregivers of children with special needs to care for these children in the home setting.

The cost of the handbook was minimal. However, it was a very effective marketing tool. Families and referral sources loved it and we were constantly complimented on providing this free to parents and family members.

We also developed a handbook for Home IV Therapy and other procedures. When we participated in Health Fairs or Seniors Events, we placed our training guides on display along with our brochures and newsletters. (See samples)

Our staff loved the fact that we provided this material to patients and families and it really helped us develop the reputation of being professional and committed to being an education-oriented care provider.

HOME IV TEACHING MANUAL SAMPLE

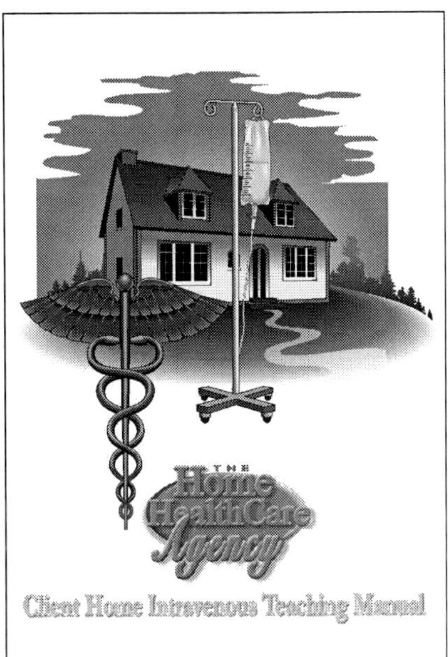

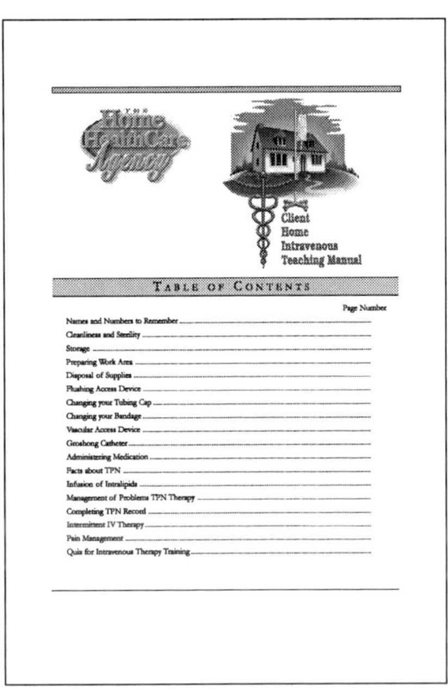

TABLE OF CONTENTS

IMPORTANT NAMES AND NUMBERS TO REMEMBER

Partners Home Health Telephone Number: ....

Your Partners Home Health Nurse is: ....

Your Partners Home Health Pharmacist is: ....

Physician: ....

Phone: ....

Paramedics: ....

Other Instructions: ....

STERILITY

INTRODUCTION

Based on your unique individual needs, your physician has determined the proper therapy for you and will continue to direct your care at home. Under your physician's direction, the Partners Home Health Inc. nurses and pharmacists will assist in your home therapy.

This manual has been developed to teach you how to manage your home therapy once you leave the hospital. With the guidance of this material and the assistance of qualified medical personnel, you will learn a safe and effective method of administering your therapy. In order to meet your individual needs, Partners Home Health Inc. has assembled the specific information you will require. Included in this manual are the following sections:

- **Cleanliness and Sterility**
- **Storing Your Drugs and Supplies**
- **Preparing Your Work Area**
- **Disposal of Medical Waste**
- **Flushing Your Access Device**
- **Changing Your Tubing Cap**
- **Changing Your Bandage**
- **Your Access Device**
  - ☐ Peripheral Catheter
  - ☐ Hickman/Broviac Catheter
  - ☐ Infusion Port
  - ☐ Groshong Catheter
  - ☐ Peripherally Inserted Central Catheter
- **Administering Your Prescribed Medication**
  - ☐ Gravity
  - ☐ Infusion Device Instruction
- **Monitoring Your Progress**
  - ☐ Total Parenteral Nutrition
  - ☐ Intermittent Therapy
  - ☐ Pain Management
- **Potential Complications**

You and your instructor will follow these "learning steps" in each section of the manual:

1. You will read the sections prior to your learning session.
2. Your instructor will review the section with you.
3. Your instructor will demonstrate the procedure to you.
4. You will repeat the procedure for your instructor.
5. When you are ready, you will start performing your own care under the direction of your instructor.

At all times, you should feel free to ask questions. You will be responsible for your care at home so it is of utmost importance that you thoroughly understand each area of your therapy. For success you must perform the procedures exactly as you have been instructed. Partners Home Health Inc. is dedicated to helping you achieve success with your therapy.

CLEANLINESS & STERILITY

In preparation for home therapy, a small tube (catheter) or port has been inserted into your body. The tube or port is called your Access Device. The access device will allow the medication to be delivered directly into your blood stream or other body part.

Cleanliness is the term used to describe the many steps you will be taught to keep your access device free from infection. It is important to remember that many normal germs which are harmless on your skin or in your mouth, can cause severe infection if they reach the inside of your body.

In order to avoid infection, you must prevent all contact between your access device and any dirt or invisible germs. To maintain cleanliness, you'll need to pay strict attention to your access device, your work area, the storage methods of drugs and all other supplies.

Sterile is a term that means absolutely free from all germs. Your hands and skin will never be sterile, as some germs are always normally present, even after thorough washing. Anything that directly touches or connects to your access device must be sterile. For this reason, many of your supplies will be delivered in sterile packages, and you will be taught not to touch the connectors, even with clean hands.
To maintain sterility, follow these steps:

1. **Wash your hands** before opening the sterile supplies.
2. **Do not** use any solution after the expiration date.

HOME IV TEACHING MANUAL SAMPLE CONTINUED

Sterility

3. **Inspect all** bottles/bags for visible signs of contamination such as cracks, chips, tears, cloudiness, discoloration, leaks, damaged caps, or solids floating in the solution.
4. **Make sure** that all packages are sealed. Inspect the tubing, needles, syringes and prep pads. Discard anything with a broken seal. If there is moisture inside the packages of tubing, needles, or syringes, discard the item.
5. **Do not** let the outside of the package touch the item inside.
6. **Do not** touch any sterile item with your fingers. Do not let the item touch any nonsterile surface.
7. After removing protective caps, **do not touch** the ends of the tubing, tubing spikes, or needles with your fingers or allow them to touch any nonsterile surface.
8. **Do not touch** the end of the access device with your fingers or allow it to touch any nonsterile surface.
9. **Do not touch** the skin around your access site with your fingers.
10. **Do not touch** the syringe plunger shaft with your fingers.
11. ***When in doubt, throw it away.***

Following these techniques is very important

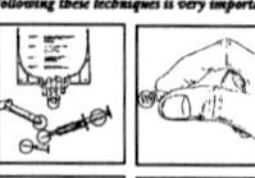

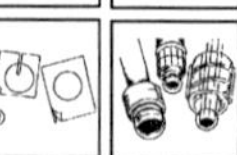

Handwashing

Thorough handwashing is included as a step prior to all your procedures. Invisible germs on your hands are the most common cause of infection.

1. Perform all "dirty" procedures like opening shipping carton, **before** washing your hands.
2. Turn on water and regulate temperature. You will leave the water running throughout the procedure.
3. Wet your hands and forearms under the running water.

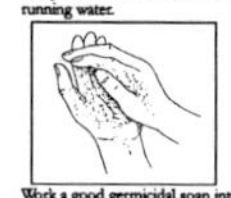

4. Work a good germicidal soap into a lather. Keep your hands down and beginning with your fingertips, move upwards to your forearms. Rub vigorously for approximately 1-2 minutes. **Don't forget to wash thoroughly between your fingers and under your fingernails.**
5. Rinse hands thoroughly under running water.
6. Dry your hands well with a paper towel or clean hand towel.

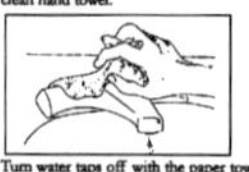

7. Turn water taps off with the paper towel or hand towel.
8. Discard paper towel or put hand towel in to be washed.

Storage

Storing Your Drug Solutions

A Home HealthCare Agency. staff person will ensure that your drug is delivered on a regular basis and help you arrange for appropriate storage. Depending on the physician and pharmacist's recommendation, the drug may be delivered frozen, refrigerated or at room temperature. The following information will help you store your drugs safely.

Warning

Regardless of whether your drug is frozen, refrigerated or stored at room temperature, notify your nurse and **DO NOT use the drug if:**

1. It has passed the expiration date.
2. It is not labeled with your name.
3. It is leaking or damaged in any manner.
4. It appears cloudy or contains floating particles.

As a final precaution, be sure all drugs and supplies are stored away from small children.

Storing Your Drug Solutions

Frozen Drugs

1. Your freezer should be able to maintain a temperature of approximately -4°F (-20°C).
2. The drug will be delivered in individual containers. Remove one sealed container from the freezer _____hours prior to administration. When thawing, place the drug in an area protected from extreme heat and light.
3. Do not force thaw by using water baths or other sources of external heat, like a microwave oven.
4. Thawed drugs should NOT be refrozen.
5. Thawed drugs should be used within 24 hours after they have been thawed.
6. Check the expiration dates; always use the oldest drugs first.

Refrigerated Drugs

1. The refrigerator should be able to maintain a temperature of approximately 40°-46°F (4°C 7°C).
2. Remove the drug from the refrigerator _____ hours prior to administration. Remove only the drugs you intend to use immediately.
3. Warm the refrigerated drugs at room temperature (70°-74°F) for _____ hours in an area protected from extreme heat and light.
4. DO NOT warm the drug by using water baths or other sources of external heat, like a microwave oven.
5. When the drug is removed from the refrigerator, it MUST be used within 24 hours. If this is not done, medication MUST be discarded.
6. Check the expiration dates; always use the oldest drug first.

Room Temperature Drugs

1. Store your drugs in a clean, cool, dark area, separate from other household supplies.
2. Check the expiration dates; always use the oldest drug first.

Preparing Your Work Area and Supplies

1. **Select a clean work area.** This area should be free of dust and drafts and away from household traffic, especially children and pets. You should also choose an area that would most likely have the fewest number of germs. Avoid using the washroom if at all possible.

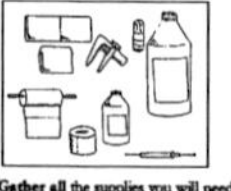

2. **Gather all** the supplies you will need for your procedure.

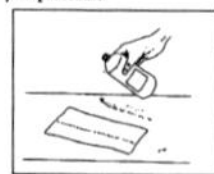

Waste Disposal

3. **Wipe down** your work area with 1:10 bleach solution and a paper towel.
4. **Do not** talk, sneeze or cough directly over your work area. Turn your head away should any of these actions be necessary.
5. **Inspect all** drugs and supplies for cracks, damaged caps and/or particles before use. Discard any defective materials.
6. Make certain that items are **clean and sterile** before use. Discard any opened, soiled or wet items. WHEN IN DOUBT OF THE CLEANLINESS OF ANY ITEM, DO NOT USE IT; CALL YOUR NURSE.
7. **Wash your hands.**
8. When opening sterile packages or removing protective caps **avoid touching** the inside with fingers, clothing or any items which may contain germs.
9. **Wipe** entry area of any drug container with an alcohol wipe to kill any germs which might be present. Do not touch these surfaces once you have swabbed them. Allow them to dry before using.

Disposal of Supplies

Just as there are germs normally present on your hands and skin, there can be normal germs within your body. To avoid contact with these germs, by yourself and others, it is important to dispose of your supplies correctly.

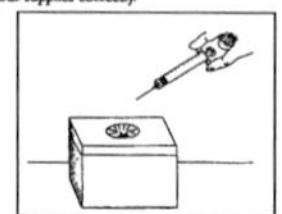

All needles and syringes should be placed in the special red "sharps" box or a hard plastic or metal container with lid. Any remaining drug solutions, the drug container and tubing should be disposed of as you have been instructed.

According to policy, Partners Home Health must pick up your "sharps" container and dispose of it according to the requirements of Federal and state requirements as long as you are a patient of ours. Again, remember to keep all drugs, needles and supplies in a safe place, away from small children.

Flushing

Flushing Your Access Device

In order to prevent clotting in the access device, and to push all medication or solution into your body, you will need to flush your access device. Flush your access device with

____________________solution

every____________________.

How to Flush Your Access Device

1. **Gather supplies** needed:
   - ☐ Bottles(s) of flushing solution
   - ☐ _____ size syringes
   - ☐ _____ size needles
   - ☐ Three Betadine swabs
2. **Wash hands** thoroughly for 1 minute.
3. **Rub top** of flush solution bottle(s) with Betadine swab for 1 minute. DO NOT touch the top of the bottle with your finger.
4. **Remove** needle cover and draw back _____ ml. of air. **DO NOT TOUCH** the needle or plunger shaft.
5. **Insert needle** with syringe into flush solution bottle.
6. Hold flush solution bottle **upside down**; push air into bottle.
7. Now **pull back** on plunger until you have drawn up the correct amount of flush solution. Remove needle from flush solution bottle.

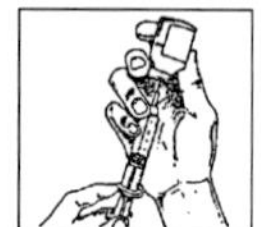

8. **Holding syringe** with needle pointing up, tap barrel with finger to move any air bubbles to the top. Expel air by gently pushing up on the plunger until a drop of solution appears at the tip of the needle. Replace needle cover.

9. **Place** solution-filled syringe in a clean, safe, convenient place.
10. **Rub** rubber stopper on tubing carefully for 2 minutes with two Betadine swabs (one minute with each swab).

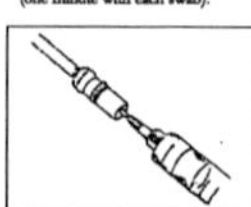

11. **Remove cover** from solution needle.
12. **Insert needle** straight into center of rubber stopper. If you are using a clamp, remove it.
13. **Slowly inject** solution and then remove needle.
14. If flush solution cannot be injected, your access device may be clotted. **Do not force solution into your access device.** Notify your nurse of the problem immediately.

Cap Change

Changing Your Tubing Cap

It is important to change the cap on the tubing which enters your body on a regular basis. This cap is actually a self-sealing rubber stopper, and during normal procedures, is punctured by needles and other devices. After a number of uses, the cap will no longer seal. To prevent this problem, your tubing cap will be change

____________________times a week.

To change the cap:

1. **Gather supplies:**
   - ☐ Tubing cap
   - ☐ Betadine wipes
   - ☐ Alcohol wipe
   - ☐ Catheter clamp
   - ☐ Tape
   - ☐ Syringe with saline
2. **Wash hands** thoroughly for 1 minute.
3. **Open** Betadine and alcohol swabs.
4. **Open** the package with cap. Do not touch the cap.

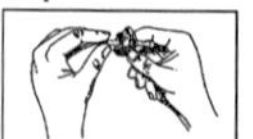

5. **Flush** the new cap with saline to remove all air.
6. Clean the connection between the tubing and the old cap with 2 Betadine swabs for 1 minute each.
7. If you've been instructed to use a clamp, use it now to **clamp** the tube. Remember to clamp the tube in a **different place** each time.
8. **Place** an alcohol wipe around the old tubing cap and the tube.
9. **Remove** the old cap.

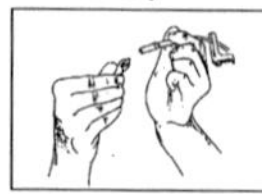

10. **Pick up** the new cap, being careful not to touch the park of the cap that will go inside the tube. Screw on the new cap securely, but be careful not to screw it on too tight.
11. If you have clamped the tube, **remove** the clamp.
12. **Tape** the connection between the cap and the tube.
13. Now **Flush** your tube as you have been instructed.

PEDIATRIC HOME HEALTH GUIDE SAMPLE

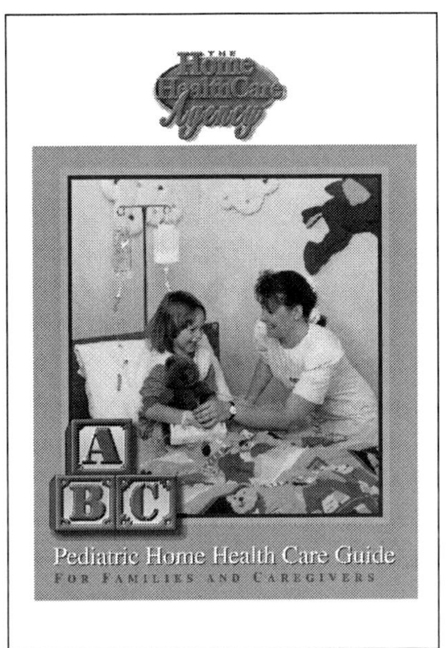

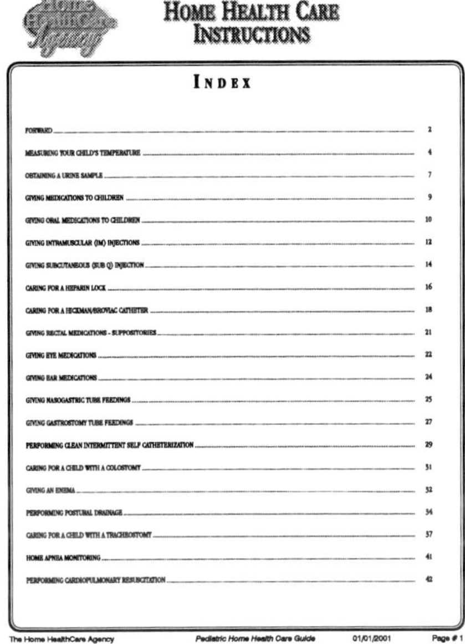

HOME HEALTH CARE INSTRUCTIONS

INDEX

The Home HealthCare Agency *Pediatric Home Health Care Guide* 01/01/2001 Page # 1

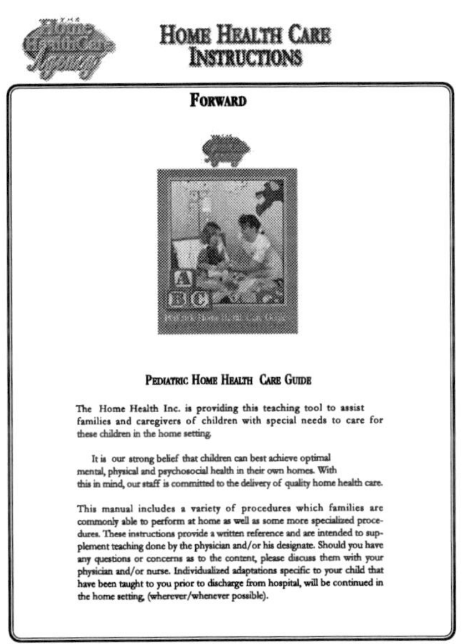

HOME HEALTH CARE INSTRUCTIONS

FORWARD

PEDIATRIC HOME HEALTH CARE GUIDE

The Home Health Inc. is providing this teaching tool to assist families and caregivers of children with special needs to care for these children in the home setting.

It is our strong belief that children can best achieve optimal mental, physical and psychosocial health in their own homes. With this in mind, our staff is committed to the delivery of quality home health care.

This manual includes a variety of procedures which families are commonly able to perform at home as well as some more specialized procedures. These instructions provide a written reference and are intended to supplement teaching done by the physician and/or his designate. Should you have any questions or concerns as to the content, please discuss them with your physician and/or nurse. Individualized adaptations specific to your child that have been taught to you prior to discharge from hospital, will be continued in the home setting, (wherever/whenever possible).

The Home HealthCare Agency *Pediatric Home Health Care Guide* 01/01/2001 Page # 2

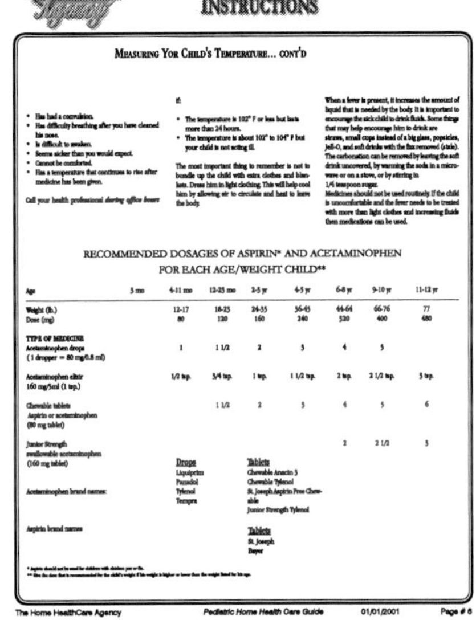

HOME HEALTH CARE INSTRUCTIONS

MEASURING YOR CHILD'S TEMPERATURE... CONT'D

- Has had a convulsion.
- Has difficulty breathing after you have cleaned his nose.
- Is difficult to awaken.
- Seems sicker than you would expect.
- Cannot be comforted.
- Has a temperature that continues to rise after medicine has been given.

Call your health professional *during office hours* if:

- The temperature is 102° F or less but lasts more than 24 hours.
- The temperature is about 102° to 104° F but your child is not acting ill.

The most important thing to remember is not to bundle up the child with extra clothes and blankets. Dress him in light clothing. This will help cool him by allowing air to circulate and heat to leave the body.

When a fever is present, it increases the amount of liquid that is needed by the body. It is important to encourage the sick child to drink fluids. Some things that may help encourage him to drink are straws, small cups instead of a big glass, popsicles, Jell-O, and soft drinks with the fizz removed (stale). The carbonation can be removed by leaving the soft drink uncovered, by warming the soda in a microwave or on a stove, or by stirring in 1/4 teaspoon sugar.
Medicines should not be used routinely. If the child is uncomfortable and the fever needs to be treated with more than light clothes and increasing fluids then medications can be used.

RECOMMENDED DOSAGES OF ASPIRIN* AND ACETAMINOPHEN FOR EACH AGE/WEIGHT CHILD**

Age	3 mo	4-11 mo	12-23 mo	2-3 yr	4-5 yr	6-8 yr	9-10 yr	11-12 yr
Weight (lb.)		12-17	18-23	24-35	36-45	44-64	66-76	77
Dose (mg)		80	120	160	240	320	400	480
TYPE OF MEDICINE								
Acetaminophen drops (1 dropper = 80 mg/0.8 ml)		1	1 1/2	2	3	4	5	
Acetaminophen elixir 160 mg/5ml (1 tsp.)		1/2 tsp.	3/4 tsp.	1 tsp.	1 1/2 tsp.	2 tsp.	2 1/2 tsp.	3 tsp.
Chewable tablets Aspirin or acetaminophen (80 mg tablet)			1 1/2	2	3	4	5	6
Junior Strength swallowable acetaminophen (160 mg tablet)						2	2 1/2	3

Acetaminophen brand names:
Drops: Liquiprim, Panadol, Tylenol, Tempra
Tablets: Chewable Anacin 3, Chewable Tylenol, St. Joseph Aspirin Free Chewable, Junior Strength Tylenol

Aspirin brand names
Tablets: St. Joseph, Bayer

* Aspirin should not be used for children with chicken pox or flu.
** [illegible]

The Home HealthCare Agency *Pediatric Home Health Care Guide* 01/01/2001 Page # 6

PEDIATRIC HOME HEALTH GUIDE SAMPLE CONTINUED

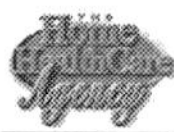

HOME HEALTH CARE INSTRUCTIONS

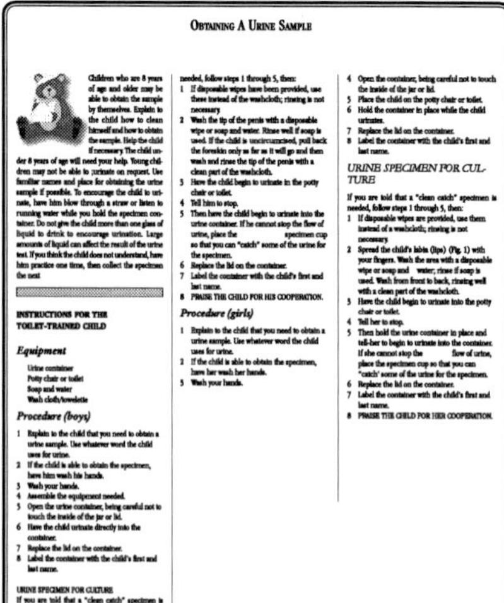

OBTAINING A URINE SAMPLE

Children who are 8 years of age and older may be able to obtain the sample by themselves. Explain to the child how to clean himself and how to obtain the sample. Help the child if necessary. The child under 8 years of age will need your help. Young children may not be able to ;urinate on request. Use familiar names and place for obtaining the urine sample if possible. To encourage the child to urinate, have him blow through a straw or listen to running water while you hold the specimen container. Do not give the child more than one glass of liquid to drink to encourage urination. Large amounts of liquid can affect the result of the urine test. If you think the child does not understand, have him practice one time, then collect the specimen the next

INSTRUCTIONS FOR THE TOILET-TRAINED CHILD

Equipment

Urine container
Potty chair or toilet
Soap and water
Wash cloth/towelette

Procedure (boys)

1 Explain to the child that you need to obtain a urine sample. Use whatever word the child uses for urine.
2 If the child is able to obtain the specimen, have him wash his hands.
3 Wash your hands.
4 Assemble the equipment needed.
5 Open the urine container, being careful not to touch the inside of the jar or lid.
6 Have the child urinate directly into the container.
7 Replace the lid on the container.
8 Label the container with the child's first and last name.

URINE SPECIMEN FOR CULTURE

If you are told that a "clean catch" specimen is needed, follow steps 1 through 5, then:

1 If disposable wipes have been provided, use these instead of the washcloth; rinsing is not necessary.
2 Wash the tip of the penis with a disposable wipe or soap and water. Rinse well if soap is used. If the child is uncircumcised, pull back the foreskin only as far as it will go and then wash and rinse the tip of the penis with a clean part of the washcloth.
3 Have the child begin to urinate in the potty chair or toilet.
4 Tell him to stop.
5 Then have the child begin to urinate into the urine container. If he cannot stop the flow of urine, place the specimen cup so that you can "catch" some of the urine for the specimen.
6 Replace the lid on the container.
7 Label the container with the child's first and last name.
8 PRAISE THE CHILD FOR HIS COOPERATION.

Procedure (girls)

1 Explain to the child that you need to obtain a urine sample. Use whatever word the child uses for urine.
2 If the child is able to obtain the specimen, have her wash her hands.
3 Wash your hands.
4 Open the container, being careful not to touch the inside of the jar or lid.
5 Place the child on the potty chair or toilet.
6 Hold the container in place while the child urinates.
7 Replace the lid on the container.
8 Label the container with the child's first and last name.

URINE SPECIMEN FOR CULTURE

If you are told that a "clean catch" specimen is needed, follow steps 1 through 5, then:

1 If disposable wipes are provided, use them instead of a washcloth; rinsing is not necessary.
2 Spread the child's labia (lips) (Fig. 1) with your fingers. Wash the area with a disposable wipe or soap and water; rinse if soap is used. Wash from front to back, rinsing well with a clean part of the washcloth.
3 Have the child begin to urinate into the potty chair or toilet.
4 Tell her to stop.
5 Then hold the urine container in place and tell her to begin to urinate into the container. If she cannot stop the flow of urine, place the specimen cup so that you can "catch" some of the urine for the specimen.
6 Replace the lid on the container.
7 Label the container with the child's first and last name.
8 PRAISE THE CHILD FOR HER COOPERATION.

The Home HealthCare Agency | *Pediatric Home Health Care Guide* | 01/01/2001 | Page # 7

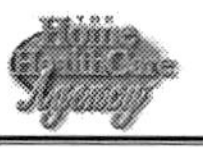

HOME HEALTH CARE INSTRUCTIONS

PLEASE READ THIS

Changes in the health care system are prompting early discharge from both acute care and home health agencies. With increasing frequency, families are being asked to provide specialized care for a child at home. Unit S presents Home Health Care Instructions (HCI) that can be used as a guide while the family is learning the procedure and then as a reference when the family performs the procedure in the absence of the health professional. The HCI should be an integral part of discharge planning to prepare the family to safely and competently care for the child at home.

This unit includes a variety of procedures that families are commonly asked to perform at home as more specialized procedures.

PREPARING THE FAMILY FOR HOME CARE

The Home Care Instructions (HCI) in this unit are provided as a supplement to assist the nurse in preparing the family to manage the child's care at home. These instructions provide a written reference that the family can use when performing the procedure in the absence of a health professional.
The HCI can be used as a teaching aid in preparing the patient for discharge from an acute care setting, or in the home when increasing the family's participation in the child's care.
The process of patient education involves giving the family information about the child's condition, the regimen that must be followed, and other health teaching as indicated. The goal of this education is to enable the family to modify behaviors and adhere to the regimen that has been mutually established.
One common problem with patient education is that the health professional delivers the information and the family listens. This one-way flow of material may not achieve the goal of the education. It is estimated that there is only a 50% compliance rate following patient education. Research has also shown that if the family is provided written information that they can understand, they are more likely to comply with the regimen.
To maximize the benefits of patient teaching, these guidelines should be followed:

1. Establish a rapport with the family.
2. Avoid using any jargon. Clarify all terms with the family.
3. When possible, allow the family to decide how they want to be taught, for example, all at once or over a day or two. This gives the family a chance to incorporate the information at a rate that is comfortable.
4. Teach the family about the illness.
5. Assist the family in identifying obstacles in their ability to comply with the regimen and the means to overcome those obstacles. Then help the family find ways to incorporate the regimen into their daily lives.

HOW TO USE THE HCI

Thoroughly review the HCI that will be given to the family. Make two photocopies, one for the family and one to attach to the nursing care plan. Fill in any blanks and individualize the instructions as necessary. If equipment will be needed at home (for example, suction machines or syringes), begin making the necessary arrangements so that discharge can proceed smoothly. Whenever possible, make arrangements for the family to use the same equipment in the home that they are using in the hospital. This allows them to become familiar with the items; in addition the staff can help "troubleshoot" the equipment in a controlled environment. When the family is being taught at home, individualize the instructions and include any adaptations that will be necessary for the family. Plan the teaching sessions well in advance of the time the family will be responsible for performing the care. The more complex the procedure, the more time is needed.
Review the instructions with the family. Allow ample practice time under supervision. At least one family member, but preferably two members, should demonstrate or discuss the care before they are expected to care for the child at home. Provide the family with the telephone numbers of resource individuals who are available to assist them in the event of a problem.

The Home HealthCare Agency | *Pediatric Home Health Care Guide* | 01/01/2001 | Page # 3

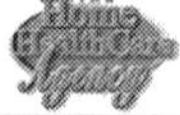

HOME HEALTH CARE INSTRUCTIONS

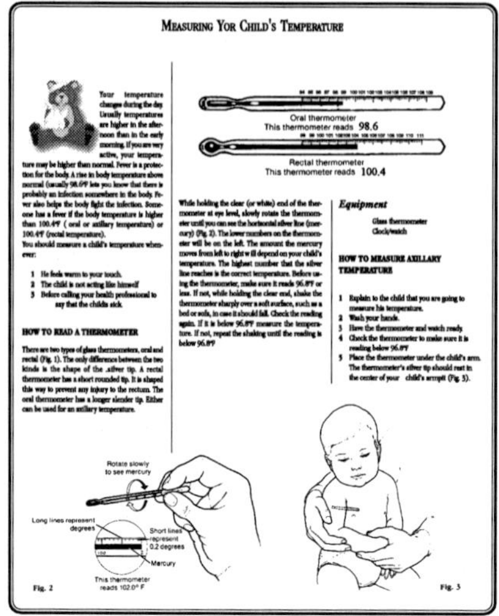

MEASURING YOR CHILD'S TEMPERATURE

Your temperature changes during the day. Usually temperatures are higher in the afternoon than in the early morning. If you are very active, your temperature may be higher than normal. Fever is a protection for the body. A rise in body temperature above normal (usually 98.6°F) lets you know that there is probably an infection somewhere in the body. Fever also helps the body fight the infection. Someone has a fever if the body temperature is higher than 100.4°F (oral or axillary temperature) or 100.4°F (rectal temperature).
You should measure a child's temperature whenever:

1 He feels warm to your touch.
2 The child is not acting like himself
3 Before calling your health professional to say that the childis sick.

HOW TO READ A THERMOMETER

There are two types of glass thermometers, oral and rectal (Fig. 1). The only difference between the two kinds is the shape of the .silver tip. A rectal thermometer has a short rounded tip. It is shaped this way to prevent any injury to the rectum. The oral thermometer has a longer slender tip. Either can be used for an axillary temperature.

While holding the clear (or white) end of the thermometer at eye level, slowly rotate the thermometer until you can see the horizontal silver line (mercury) (Fig. 2). The lower numbers on the thermometer will be on the left. The amount the mercury moves from left to right will depend on your child's temperature. The highest number that the silver line reaches is the correct temperature. Before using the thermometer, make sure it reads 96.8°F or less. If not, while holding the clear end, shake the thermometer sharply over a soft surface, such as a bed or sofa, in case it should fall. Check the reading again. If it is below 96.8°F measure the temperature. If not, repeat the shaking until the reading is below 96.8°F

Equipment

Glass thermometer
Clock/watch

HOW TO MEASURE AXILLARY TEMPERATURE

1 Explain to the child that you are going to measure his temperature.
2 Wash your hands.
3 Have the thermometer and watch ready.
4 Check the thermometer to make sure it is reading below 96.8°F
5 Place the thermometer under the child's arm. The thermometer's silver tip should rest in the center of your child's armpit (Fig. 3).

Fig. 2

Fig. 3

The Home HealthCare Agency | *Pediatric Home Health Care Guide* | 01/01/2001 | Page # 4

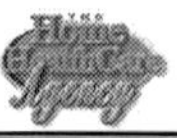

HOME HEALTH CARE INSTRUCTIONS

MEASURING YOR CHILD'S TEMPERATURE...CONT'D

6 Hold the child's arm firmly against his body.
7 Check the time.
8 The thermometer must remain in place for 3 to 4 minutes. This may seem like a long time. To help make the time seem to go faster, read a story or watch television with the child. Make sure you hold the thermometer securely.
9 Remove the thermometer and read the temperature.
10 Write down the thermometer reading and the time of day.

HOW TO MEASURE RECTAL TEMPERATURES

Note that rectal temperatures should not be taken if the child has diarrhea or is less than 1 year old. In taking a child's temperature rectally, use the following procedure:

1 Explain to the child that you will be measuring his temperature.
2 Wash your hands.
3 Have the thermometer and watch ready (and a clean diaper if needed).
4 Check to make sure that the thermometer is reading less than 96.8°F
5 Measure 1 inch on the thermometer or approximately 1/6 of the thermometers length.
6 Place the child on his stomach, on one side with the upper leg bent, or on back with both legs up (Fig. 4).
7 Dip the thermometer s silver tip in a lubricant such as petroleum jelly (Vaseline).
8 Place the silver end of the thermometer into the child's anus.
9 Do not insert the thermometer any further than 1 inch.
10 Check the time.
11 Hold the thermometer in place for 2 to 3 minutes. Always hold the child so that he cannot twist around.
12 Remove thermometer and read.
13 Write down the thermometer reading and the time of day.

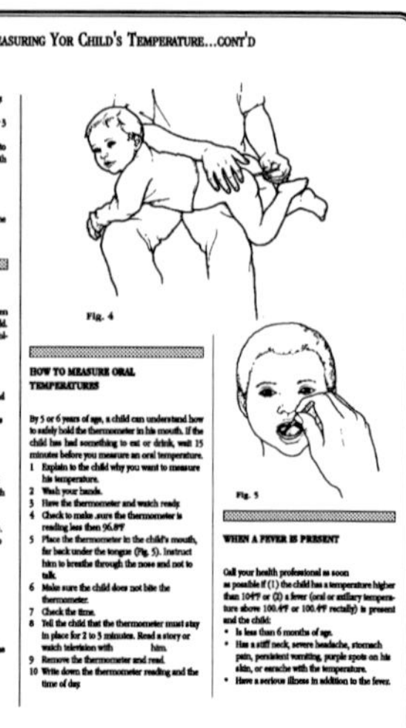

Fig. 4

Fig. 5

HOW TO MEASURE ORAL TEMPERATURES

By 5 or 6 years of age, a child can understand how to safely hold the thermometer in his mouth. If the child has had something to eat or drink, wait 15 minutes before you measure an oral temperature.

1 Explain to the child why you want to measure his temperature.
2 Wash your hands.
3 Have the thermometer and watch ready.
4 Check to make .sure the thermometer is reading less then 96.8°F
5 Place the thermometer in the child's mouth, far back under the tongue (Fig. 5). Instruct him to breathe through the nose and not to talk.
6 Make sure the child does not bite the thermometer.
7 Check the time.
8 Tell the child that the thermometer must stay in place for 2 to 3 minutes. Read a story or watch television with him.
9 Remove the thermometer and read.
10 Write down the thermometer reading and the time of day.

WHEN A FEVER IS PRESENT

Call your health professional as soon as possible if (1) the child has a temperature higher than 104°F or (2) a fever (oral or axillary temperature above 100.4°F or 100.4°F rectally) is present and the child:

- Is less than 6 months of age.
- Has a stiff neck, severe headache, stomach pain, persistent vomiting, purple spots on his skin, or earache with the temperature.
- Have a serious illness in addition to the fever.

The Home HealthCare Agency | *Pediatric Home Health Care Guide* | 01/01/2001 | Page # 5

CHAPTER FORTY-ONE

Monthly Newsletter

Advertising is nothing more than salesmanship in print.

— John E. Kennedy

One of the best ways to market your agency is to educate, inform and service your prospects and existing clients. The single best marketing tool is the newsletter.

The Power of Having a Monthly Newsletter

A "client newsletter" can be one of the most powerful tools for maintaining relationships with your clients, keeping them interested in your agency and your services. A monthly newsletter can also be used as a great sales tool for prospective clients.

- It develops a relationship between your agency and your client. A monthly newsletter is a very easy and inexpensive way of keeping in constant contact with your clients. Your newsletter has a better chance of getting read by a decision maker because newsletters are put in the same category as magazines, newspapers and trade journals. They get more respect from the "gate keeper" and are more apt to be read.

- It keeps your agency "in front of" your clients. Remember — every month you don't contact a client you lose 10% of the value of your relationship. Thus, if you don't contact your client for 10 months... the relationship is over.
- It gives your agency an opportunity to up-sell your existing clients and introduce new services.
- Your agency can recognize clients who have referred others to you. By recognizing these clients they will want to continue referring new clients to your agency. In addition, existing clients will want to refer because they will read how others are already doing it.

The Look of Your Newsletter

Your newsletter should have a consistent look each month. I recommend developing a template for your newsletter consisting of a masthead (top partor side bar of the first page), headline type, boxes and borders. You can have a professional design the overall look of your newsletter (with logo, masthead, etc.) and have it supplied on a disc — for you or your print vendor. Once you have the template established, all you have to do is insert the new copy and illustrations.

Your newsletter should be well designed and easy to read, with 2, 4, or 8 single-spaced typeset pages. Include photographs and illustrations with text at every opportunity, i.e. nurses of the month, new staff, etc.

Content Tips for Newsletters

Putting your message into a publication in the context of an article gets better readership than "sales material" and "ads" — so it makes sense to put your information and message into publication. Using an article format, such as in a newsletter, adds a "personal touch feeling" and will increase the readership of your marketing message to clients and prospects.

Keep articles short, less than one page. Proof copy carefully — you don't want to be embarrassed by improper grammar and spelling errors.

Content for your newsletter could include:

- Letter from the president
- Information/education directly linked to your service
- Client recognition and appreciation
- Birthdays
- Referrals
- Testimonials
- Promotion of new services
- Requests for Referrals
- Health tips
- "Meet the Staff" articles
- "Meet the Clients" articles
- Common dilemmas with solutions that your clients can relate to.
- General area news and events

Encourage your clients to call or write to you with comments and/or suggestions for future newsletters. This will help to build strong relationships between you and your clients and maintain a dialogue between your agency and clients.

Who writes your newsletter?

You do!

No one knows your agency better than you and your staff. Don't hire another firm to write impersonal and generic copy about your agency. Find the time each month to write interesting, informative, friendly copy that your clients and prospects will appreciate. A poorly written, poorly designed newsletter can have a negative affect on your agency — it would be better to scrap the idea altogether. Spend the time each month to produce a quality newsletter — even if it is only a 2-page newsletter — and the results will be incredible!

Write the newsletter in a one-on-one style. Avoid formality and being too impersonal — keep it friendly. Write your newsletter as if your reader is sitting across from you and you are telling him or her what's going on in your agency (such as new services, new nurses, success stories about other clients, how your agency has helped or solved a dilemma, etc.).

Sending Newsletters

Your newsletter should be sent out every month like clockwork. Whether it arrives on the 15th or the 30th of each month, it's important that your newsletter be there when the reader expects it.

If you set up your newsletter as a "self-mailer" with an area for the address, you can do away with stuffing envelopes. Also if you have a large database (list), I suggest getting a bulk-rate mailing indicia for your newsletters. This will save you approximately 30–40% on postage for each mailing. You can get it at your local post office in the bulk rate department.

If you decide to put your newsletter into an envelope, keep the envelope personal looking.

- Always use real stamps.
- Use labels that draw the eye or **hand write** the address.

Your newsletter can be sent to hospitals, trustees, discharge nurses, physicians, etc. Newsletters help to develop a sense of community with your clients and encourage word-of-mouth referrals.

- Clients
- Prospects and Referrals
- Referral Sources
- Tradeshow visitors
- Primary family members of clients

Courtesy Newsletters

I encourage your agency to send "courtesy newsletters" to prospective clients. From your newsletters, they will learn of your services, read testimonials of happy clients, and get a sense of your care style and personal approach. When they do make a Home Care service decision, they will be more likely to hire your agency.

When sending a courtesy newsletter, always attach a cover letter. The following is an example of a cover sheet that I recommend using.

Dear Susan Davis,

My name is Sally Wilson. I am a home care administrator for (Your Company Name), a home care provider in your community. Our agency has assisted a substantial number of local clients with their health concerns, daily life challenges, and overall care. Our goal is to enhance the quality of life for every client we serve.

We also publish our own newsletter for our family of clients and staff with up-todate information on health issues, as well articles on our own outreach and expanding services. We enjoy sharing our newsletter and try to keep it interesting and helpful.

I don't know if our agency could assist you, but I thought you might enjoy receiving a few copies of our newsletter. I have arranged to send you a copy with my compliments for the next three months. It is our way of introducing ourselves to you — and we certainly hope you find it informative and useful.

If you feel that I could be of service to you, I would be happy to meet with you for a free consultation to discuss your particular situation. Please feel free to call me at 1-555-555-5555 to arrange an appointment.

Our agency also has several free brochures and informative health care related reports that might be of interest to you. I've listed them on the enclosed card. If you fill out the card and send it back, I will put the information in the mail to you right away.

Please enjoy the newsletters and let me know if we can assist you or a loved one in any way in the future.

Sincerely,

Sally Wilson
Administrator
The Home Care Agency

After receiving your newsletter for a few months, clients and prospects will not only come to expect it, they look forward to receiving it. Readers know they'll learn from it. They will respect your agency, and many prospects will eventually become clients.

Sending a monthly newsletter to your clients is a must. It is necessary to maintain your existing clients. (See sample newsletter)

Please feel free to call our office to find out how we can help you put together a monthly newsletter: 1–866–ADAMGRP.

COMPANY NEWSLETTER SAMPLE

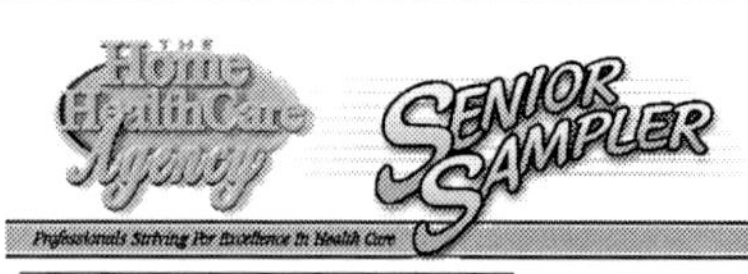

Spotlight Features

Assisted Living Resident of the Month

Our feature assisted living resident for November is Ms. Mollie Peebles. Mollie has lived at Wellington Place since October 1996. After overhearing someone talking about Wellington Place, she began to investigate and moved in. She was born in Smyrna, Tennessee, and comes from a large family with 3 brothers and 4 sisters. Her father was a farmer. Mollie worked for civil service for 30 years, and has traveled a lot in her lifetime, "from Maine to California." Mollie Says she is "an unclaimed jewel" because she has never been married. Mollie has been a joy to have at our facility. Thank you, Mollie, for being a part of our Wellington family. We appreciate the opportunity to know her and assist in her care.

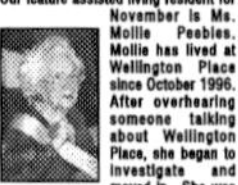

Ms. Mollie Peebles

Adult Day Care Member of the Month

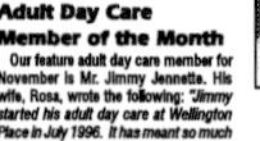

Our feature adult day care member for November is Mr. Jimmy Jennette. His wife, Rosa, wrote the following: *"Jimmy started his adult day care at Wellington Place in July 1996. It has meant so much to him to be able to interact with other people and meet new friends. He always tells me how much he has enjoyed each day he spends there. It has helped me to have a little more time at home to do things I need to do or go for appointments and know he is being cared for without having to rush back at a special time. We are so pleased to have Wellington Place in our community, and know we have friends there to help us."*

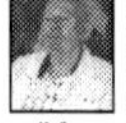

Mr. Jimmy Jennette

Jimmy has been a joy to have as a member at Wellington Place. We are glad for the opportunity to care for him, and to offer his wife this sense of security. Thank you, Jimmy, for being a part of our Wellington family.

Special Person of the Month

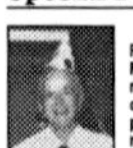

Mr. Morris Bishop

Our October Special Person of the Month, is Mr. Morris Bishop. Morris has been a member of our Adult Day Care program for about 4 months. He visits with us 3 days a week. Morris is helpful to all other members and assisted living residents. He also helps with other things around the Center. He likes to keep busy doing whatever tasks people need assistance with. Morris is also a gentleman, always holding doors open for the ladies

Morris' birthday, September 30th, was celebrated with a party in his honor. His wife wrote the following thank you note to our staff *"To all, Thank you so much for having the party for Morris. I'm sure he'll remember it for a good while. He certainly enjoyed everything. You're all so good to him.* **Sincerely, Melia."**

Morris' Favorite Poem

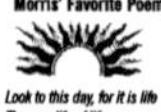

Look to this day, for it is life
The very life of life.
In its brief course
lies all the varieties and realities
of existence.
The bliss of growth
The hope of action
The glory of power.
For yesterday is but a dream.
And tomorrow is only a vision.
But today, well lived,
makes every yesterday a dream
of happiness And every tomorrow a vision of hope.
Look well, therefore, to this day!

INSIDE...

- *Construction Update*
- *Birthdays & Special Events*
- *Special Friends*
- *What Is ICMS?*
- *Employee of the Montth*
- *Health & Nutrition Tips*

Wellington Place, A GerAssist Facility

Construction Update

by Wayne Medley
Anchor Building Corp

August 1997

Construction began on the addition to Wellington Place in early July 1997 and, as of November 1st, will be 75% complete. Exterior work is just about finished, with bricks, roof, and windows already done. Interior finishing will begin the end of October. We are hopeful that the first floor hallway will be complete by the 2nd week of November, thus allowing easy access for residents to travel between buildings and avoid the cold weather.

Projected completion date is December 1st. The addition will add 17 units, 2 common areas, new patio in the existing courtyard area, drop-off canopy at the building entrance by the indoor pool, and a new building entrance. The new building addition of 8,058 square feet brings the total to 30,604 square feet under roof after completion.

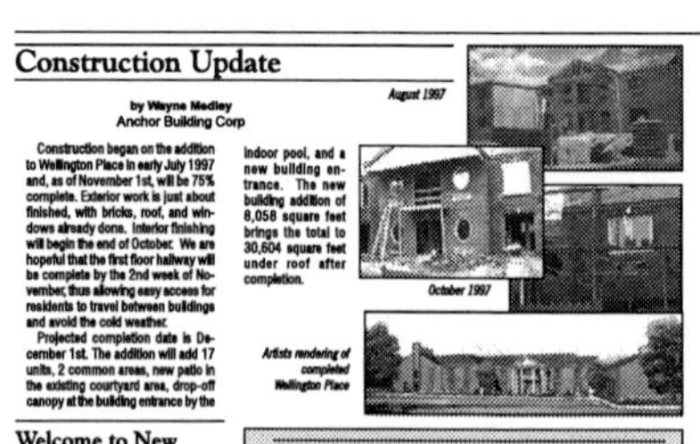

October 1997

Artists rendering of completed Wellington Place

Welcome to New Members & Residents

We want to give a warm Wellington Place welcome to Ms. Ann Watson. Ann is a new assisted living resident, now residing in Room 103. We encourage everyone to meet and welcome Ann as she makes the transition to assisted living at Wellington Place.

Special Friend of the Month

Mickey, better known as "The Ukulele Lady," visits our Center once each week. She plays songs from the 1920s, 30s, and 40s on her ukulele, and visits with all our members and residents. Everyone at Wellington Place enjoys her music, and we look forward to her visits. Thank you, Mickey, for bringing a little extra joy in our lives.

The Ukulele Lady

Special Events

All monthly activities and events are listed in our Wellington Place Activity Schedule. We will highlight special events in the Senior Sampler each month.

On Tuesday November 25th we will hoe having a Thanksgiving lunch with members and residents. Diane Gramann Director of the Integrated Care Management Center and Alzheimers Care, will present stress management tips, "Caring for Yourself," from 11:30 to 12 noon. The luncheon will follow. We hope you all will be here as we celebrate the Thanksgiving holiday together.

Caregiver Tips

by Diane Gramann
Director of ICMS

First Aid for your Mental Health

Talk it out -..... find a level headed person you can trust.
Escape for awhile -..... find a spot of peace and quiet.
Work off your anger-..... pitch into exercise or hobbies.
Give in occasionally -..... admit that you can.
Do something for others -..... it takes your mind off yourself
Take things one at a time -..... shun the "Superman" urge.
Give yourself a pat on the back for the things you do well - but don't try to be perfect.
Go easy with criticism -..... others have virtues too.
Give the other fellow a break -..... cooperation is contagious.
Make yourself available - often others are only waiting for you to make the first move.
Schedule your recreation -..... essential to good physical and mental health.
Tell someone you care.
Be able to laugh at yourself -..... and smile, smile, smile!

Courtesy of Mesa County Association for Mental Health

Page # 2 | *Wellington Place Monthly Newsletter* | *November 1997*

GerAssist Employees - Taken at Open House, November 1996

Our One Year Anniversary

Wellington Place Adult Day Health Center opened in July 1996. This consists of the Comprehensive Outpatient Rehabilitation Facility (CORF) and the Adult Day Care program. We currently have 20 members regularly attending our center. The Assisted Living Facility at Wellington Place opened in September 1996. Our Open House was held in November 1996. We currently have all 21 residents, and are looking forward to the additional 17 units being opened soon. Everyone at Wellington Place is like family, and we, as employees, are blessed to have the opportunity to serve and care for each of you. We are all looking forward to a great second year together at Wellington Place.

Employee of the Month

We at Wellington Place began selecting an Employee of the Month, with help from residents, members, and their families, in May 1997. We want to honor these employees, who have gone "above and beyond the call of duty" to touch the lives of our members and residents, in the Senior Sampler.

Employee of the Month for May 1997

The Employee of the Month for September was Ms. Shelley Holt. Shelley began working at Wellington Place in September 1996. At that time, she was a Social Work Intern. Shelley has her Bachelor's degree in Social Work from Middle Tennessee State University. Shelley enjoys her work with the residents and members, and shows a genuine interest for their wellbeing. In September 1997, Shelley was added to the staff at GerAssist's new Integrated Care Management Center, as a Care Manager Level1/ Member Services Coordinator. She will still be working with the residents and members at Wellington Place, but has expanded job responsibilities as well. We at Wellington Place want to take this opportunity to thank Shelley for her dedication and caring, and wish her well in her new role with the ICMC. • • •

Ms. Shelley Holt

Employee of the Month for October 1997

The Employee of the Month for October is Ms. Mary Teal. Mary has been with GerAssist at Wellington Place since September 1996. She works as a Care Partner at the Assisted Living facility. Mary is very hardworking and truly cares about the wellbeing of the residents she helps. She is punctual, dependable, and reliable. Mary will gladly come into work any time she's called. Thank you, Mary, for giving your best to the residents at Wellington Place. Congratulations on your one-year anniversary with our company, and we hope you are with us for many years to come.

Ms.Mary Teal

What Is ICMS?

by Diane Gramann
Director of ICMS

Integrated Care Management System (ICMS) is the newest addition to the GerAssist comprehensive senior health care company. ICMS is a system of services available to seniors throughout GerAssist that provides continuity of care to every identified member who calls or is seen at any one of our "Points of Service." Currently our points of service include Assisted Living, Home Care Services, Adult Day Care, Rehabilitation Services, and Physician Managed Services in various communities across the state from Cookeville to Memphis. As GerAssist continues to expand to better serve our customers, regional Integrated Care Management Centers (ICMC) will be located across the country. A sophisticated computer network, designed to facilitate sharing of information and enhance the care we provide to our members, will link all the ICMCs.

For more information or to become a "member" of the GerAssist Integrated Care Management System, please call 615-370-8154 or toll free 1-888-371-8171.

Delights from WP's Kitchen

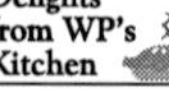

No Bake Pumpkin Cream Pie

(From Pam Johnson)

1 1/2 cup confectioners sugar
1 8-oz Package cream cheese softened
4 Tbsp. (1/2 stick) butter, softened
1 Tbsp. Vanilla
1 tsp. Pumpkin pie spice
1 16-oz can pumpkin
1 9-inch prepared graham cracker crust
1 cup heavy cream, whipped (optional)

Beat sugar, cream cheese, butter, vanilla, & pumpkin pie spice with electric mixer for 1-2 minutes, until fluffy. Add pumpkin until blended. Spoon into piecrust. Chill for 6 hours or overnight. Serve with whipped cream as desired.

November 1997 | *Wellington Place Monthly Newsletter* | *Page # 3*

From the Administrator

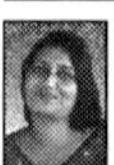

Anu Kaushal
Administrator
Wellington Place

I want to take this opportunity to welcome you all to our new Wellington Place Newsletter, the Senior Sampler. This will be a monthly publication for residents, members, and families, as well as for prospective residents and members. If you have something that you would like to have printed in future issues please feel free to bring or send it to us. This is your newsletter, and we would very much like input from each of you.

Seems like yesterday, but it's been more than a year since we welcomed our first day member and resident to Wellington Place. It's been a great year. We started with only a few members and residents, and now we have grown beyond our expectations. It is so encouraging to hear friends of Wellington say, "Everyone works like a family here." I wish I could portray every incident when I see our members, residents, and staff holding hands, walking around, singing together, dancing together, reaching out to help. All these little things which seem simple make them so special. So many times visitors say, "Everybody seems so happy here." And that is true.

All our staff work as a team to maintain an environment which has abundance of love, care, and compassion - a sincere effort to help our seniors age in place with dignity and the respect they deserve. We learn from their experiences. I would like to thank the family members of our day members and residents for giving us this opportunity to serve their loved ones — who are now our loved ones too.

Trivia Question

by Shelley Holt

"Why can't a man living south of the Ohio River be buried in his hometown?"
(Answer in next month's issue)

Health Tips

by Dr. Robert Hollister
Medical Director

Moderate Regular Exercise

It has been conclusively shown by numerous studies that daily moderate exercise, primarily walking, and/or a routine set of repetitive arm and leg motions in place and/or using one or two pound weights, will decrease body weight and increase joint mobility and decrease the pain of arthritis.

Fish Meals

A fish meal twice a week will raise the "good" cholesterol level (HDL) and lower the "bad" cholesterol level (LDL), probably due to the omega-3 fatty acid content. It will also help keep your weight under control. At the same time as we eat more fish, we need to eat less red meat.

Aspirin

An aspirin a day really does help keep the doctor away! Taking one adult aspirin tablet (5 grains) or one pediatric aspirin (1.25 grains) per day acts to decrease the tendency of blood to clot. This lowers the risk of stroke and heart attack for both men and women. If you are sensitive to aspirin or have a history of ulcers or gastritis, then a buffered or coated aspirin is recommended. Two good brands are Bufferin or Ecotrin.

Nutrition Tips

Cranberries...

tiny, red, sparkling, fiberific jewels...1 cup delivers more fiber (3.2 grams) than an equal amount of unpeeled apple slices...and yields an admirable stash of vitamin C (13 milligrams)...reportedly possesses theraputic power for the respiratory system by opening up congested bronchial tubes...and only 46 fat-free calories!

Birthdays

October 8th .... Mr. Frank Novak
October 11th ...... Ms. Pearl Vanbusleigh
October 29th .... Ms. Gladys Horton
November 8th .... Mr. Marion Davis
November 8th .... Ms. Bennie Waddell
November 13th .... Mr. Bud Ransom

Editorial Staff

And contibuting editors.

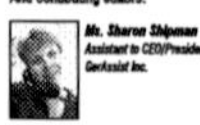

Ms. Sharon Shipman
Assistant to CEO/President
GerAssist Inc.

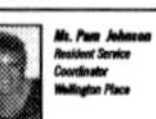

Ms. Pam Johnson
Resident Service Coordinator
Wellington Place

We endeavor to produce a publication that is informative and functional to all. We appreciate submissions and contibutions for upcoming issues.

DEADLINES:

For December Issue

All submissions to Pam or Sharon by November 14th.

Page #4 | *Wellington Place Monthly Newsletter* | *November 1997*

CHAPTER FORTY-TWO

Newspaper Column

If you would not be forgotten as soon as you are gone, either write things worth reading or do things worth writing.

— Benjamin Franklin

Another successful strategy for becoming an information source for your community is to have a newspaper column of your own. You've seen columns written by doctors, chefs and gardeners — why not home care professionals?

This day and age, with an ever increasing number of seniors and families facing the challenge of caring for their parents at home, the opportunity and need exists for your agency to have a column in the newspaper. Your column could provide informative advice, and serve as a great tool to build up community rapport and referrals.

In your column your agency would answer questions sent in by interested readers. Being able to supply written responses, through your column, provides ample time to research and address these questions and concerns.

How does your agency benefit from having a column?

First of all, when you have your own column you are considered to be the "expert" in your area.

Whenever someone in your community faces the challenge of caring for someone at home or knows someone with this challenge, they will immediately think of your agency. This is a great way to dramatically increase your business.

In addition, your agency can use excerpts from your columns in all your marketing materials, new client kits, brochures, etc. Do you think this would help your agency establish credibility? Absolutely.

How do you get a Newspaper Column?

It may take some time and persistence with the editor of the newspaper. But if you provide him/her with a letter explaining the benefits that your column could provide his/her newspaper and its readers, you will have a very good chance at running a column.

Prepare a list of column topics and actually write out a few. Determine a column word count and stay within in.
The editor will not be interested in having to take time to edit your column every week!) Show the editor that you are prepared to meet weekly deadlines. Be prepared and be persistent!

Column Topics

- What do you look for when selecting as agency?
- Benefits of home care services
- Who can qualify for home care services?
- Types of home care services available
- Respite Care
- Employment opportunities in home care
- Advice for family caregivers
- Pediatric care
- Preparing for the aging of our parents
- Alternate living choices
- Maintaining health and wellness through the aging process

CHAPTER FORTY-THREE

Publicity

What you hear repeatedly,
you will eventually believe.
— Mike Murdock

Publicity is advertising. Making sure your agency receives positive, informative publicity should be part of your marketing strategy.

The three media that can most effectively publicize your agency, your events and your services are newspapers, radio and television. How do you get publicity? Have something worth reporting.

If you are a new agency, your press releases will deal with the fact that you are new in town. If you are starting up a new service, you will want this publicized. Do you sponsor senior events? Get it in the news. Have you just hired a new nursing director? Type up a press release and send it with a photo to the papers. Are there new breakthroughs in medicine or technology that affect the Home Care industry and would interest the public? Be the first agency to get it in the news. In short, give the editors and program directors a story.

To stand out... *Stand Out!*

Word of mouth is the best publicity machine out there. But how does your name get around in the first place? Aside from clients and referral sources, public opinion can be shaped by what they see or hear in the news. People feel more comfortable when they recognize your company's name. If they read about you in the paper, they feel more comfortable calling you.

Editors and program directors for local stations are always on the lookout for compelling and useful material and news. They look to companies who come across as experts in a particular field to write articles about. Position yourself as an expert in some particular aspect of Home Care.

Several years ago our company placed ads in a weekly publication called *TV Guide*. Our ads were specifically designed to sell our support services for seniors. One day we had a call from the editor of the local newspaper asking if his paper could do a story about our company and the services we provided for seniors. The article was to run during Senior's Week. The editor told us that he had seen our ads in the *TV Guide* and decided that we must have a lot of expertise in senior care. So, when he wanted to do a story about seniors and home care services, he called us.

We called a few of our clients and asked whether they would agree to be interviewed by the paper and have their pictures taken with their caregiver. Every one of the patients we called agreed to be part of the article.

They were excited about being selected. To our surprise, the article ended up on the front page and the pictures were in color!

The response to that one article was absolutely fantastic. Within one week after the ad ran, our referrals and hours had more than doubled and continued to increase for months. We more than recovered the cost of all our weekly ads with the increased volume of new business and profit we generated from that free publicity.

Once you have established yourself as an expert and have earned a reputation of being exceptional in a particular field, find fresh ways to keep your company's name out front.

How to Write a Great Press Release… and get your agency on more radio and television talk shows.

These are the rules for writing a successful press release. If you follow these simple but proven steps you will increase your chances of getting on TV and radio by ten times.

- Press releases should be one page and one page only. If you can't tell your story in one page, the producer will think you don't know what you're talking about. There is never a good reason to have a press release go on for more than one page.
- Your press release should be on 8 1/2" x 11" paper only. Do not use odd sizes, special shapes or "original" designs.
- Your press release must be written on white paper. Do not use other colors, tints or shade color patterns.
- You must use plain white paper. No letterhead, no printed borders, no photographs. Absolutely nothing, just plain white paper.
- Never single-space the entire body copy. This is probably the number one reason press releases are thrown in the garbage by producers or show hosts.

- Use an easy-to-read typeface — no fancy fonts. "Courier" is a good choice.
- Use a catchy headline in your press release. Think of what would capture your own attention if you were on the receiving end of a press release.
- Give just the facts — who, what, when and why?
- No typos — proofread.

What goes inside the Press Release?

In the upper left corner, you're going to only have two options. You choose the one that's more appropriate for your purpose.

The first option is to put the words "For Immediate Release" in the upper left corner. These words do two things. First, they tell the producer or editor that he can use your information any time he wishes. He can use it today, tomorrow, next month, next year — whenever.

"For Immediate Release" does something even more important, though. These words tell the producer that you know how to play the publicity game. The more of these clues you can put in your release, the more confidence the producer will have in you. Keep in mind that some producers get hundreds of press releases every day. They don't have time to waste on people who don't already know how to play the "publicity game."

The only other option you have for the upper left corner is to indicate a "time qualifier." A time qualifier tells the producer exactly when and when *not* to use your release.

For example, your agency is putting together a release about a Seniors Event that is coming up. In the upper left corner you put "For Release On or Before Seniors Event." Not only are you telling the producer exactly when to use your release, you're again giving him a sign that you understand and use press "lingo." Not many press releases have time qualifiers. So if you use one the right way, you will score big points with the show producer and will increase your agency's chances of getting on the show.

In the upper right corner of your press release you only have one option. You're going to put these exact words in the upper right corner of every press release you ever write. On the first line in the upper right corner you will put: "For further information contact:" On the second line you're going to put the name and direct phone number of a real, live human being, i.e., Jane Smith — 555–555–5555.

The headline of a news release has one job and one job only — to force the producer to keep reading the rest of the copy. The headline has no other job. As mentioned earlier, write your headline so that you would find it interesting if you were reading it for the first time.

The body copy of your news release has three parts. Part One should tell your whole story in 2 or 3 sentences. If you can't tell your whole story in 2 or 3 sentences, you must practice to learn how.

Part Two of your news release should contain quotes from you along with your credentials and should expand upon the first paragraph of your news release. Always quote yourself. Never quote anyone else.

Part Three of your news release should contain your "call to action." What do you want to happen as a result of your new release?

All the time you are writing your news release, you must write in a "who cares" style of writing. That means that after every sentence you write, you should stop, read the sentence out loud and ask, "Who cares?" If you can't answer that question, you need to rethink and reword.

Once you have written your news release, the fastest way to reach newspapers, radio and local TV shows is via fax. Phone each paper or station to verify the editor or producer's name before sending a faxed press release. Verifying the contact name in advance will increase your chances of getting an interview. Then fax your release as often as possible. Everyday if you can. Be prepared to respond to same-day interviews, which can sometimes happen. Some of the smaller markets will phone you when they get your fax release.

Follow up your faxes with phone calls to the editor or show producer. Many shows get hundreds of faxed press releases per day. Help spark the producer's memory by phoning.

Don't make the mistake of thinking that press releases and free publicity won't work for your agency. In over 25 years we've never had an experience of free publicity — especially on the radio or television that we didn't benefit from. Publicity can help you get your agency started, expand it beyond anything you expected, make you a celebrity, make you an expert and make your agency the name people think of when looking for Home Care services.

CHAPTER FORTY-FOUR

Radio and TV Talk Shows

Luck is a matter of preparation meeting opportunity.

— Oprah Winfrey

When we first started our agency we sent press releases to many of the local radio stations that had older listening audiences, which were between 45–65 (children of seniors) and 65–85 (seniors). We were guests on one of the local talk radio stations talking about new services available to seniors, how they could qualify for care, and how they could apply for services. We provided valuable information to seniors with regards to the health care options available to them. This approach was extremely successful for our agency — and it was free publicity!

Television talk shows can also be a great way for your agency to get exposure on TV without having to spend thousands upon thousands of dollars. We also approached several local morning TV talk shows to see if we could be a guest on the show and talk about our agency's services and its benefits to the elderly community. The results were incredible! Our agency was immediately recognized as an expert in providing home care services to seniors in the local community and our sales and referrals dramatically increased.

In your area there are probably a few radio and TV stations with at least one or two talk shows on their daily or weekly schedule. These shows are constantly looking for new, interesting guests to talk about new services and benefits available to their audience. Just about anything can qualify you as a guest: an opinion, a survey, a new service, a promotion, a charitable contribution, etc.

Tips for Getting on a Talk Show

- For radio, call the station's producer — especially when you are in a small market. Tell them who you are, that you would like to be a guest on their show, that you have a topic of interest for their listeners, and describe the services your agency provides. You may find yourself booked in a very short time. I recommend that you phone or fax your news release to morning show producers and hosts between 10:00–11:00 A.M., after their show has gone off the air. If you wait until the afternoon to call, it may be too late for you to reach them.
- For TV, send a press release to the station that hosts the talk show introducing new services available in the community. (Writing a press release is covered in Chapter 43 — *Publicity*.)
- Represent your agency as an expert in caring for seniors — to lead educational and informative discussions or actual on-air seminars for a local general or senior audience. For example, you could provide information to family members on how to care for an elderly parent or family member, or you could talk about the services that are available to seniors, etc.

- Become aware of local "community affairs" programs that focus on elderly care or senior programs that are scheduled to be on talk shows. Offer to be a guest to provide expert advice on elderly care programs.

Tips for Talk Shows

- **Be entertaining and interesting.** Your entertaining interview will influence the show host to plug your agency. Plus, the show will get higher ratings, increasing your chances of being invited back as a guest in the future.
- **Be compelling.** It is not necessary for you to be funny, but you should strive to be interesting. You are there to keep your audience glued to the program. Your secondary purpose is to create new clients for your agency.
- **Give specific, precise answers to questions** posed by the show host or someone who calls in to a call-in show. The more information you provide, the more people will respond well to what you have to offer, and want to use your agency's services.
- **Anticipate questions from hosts and listeners.** Expect to hear familiar questions and prepare answers for these questions. This will allow you to establish a comfortable, confident and easy pace for yourself.
- **Say the word "Free" in your interview.** Have brochures, newsletters or reports prepared (describing your agency's services or pertaining to the topic) that listeners can receive by calling your office. You will then obtain names and addresses of prospects to send monthly newsletters or other interesting home care related information to.

- **Don't be an infomercial** but make sure you tell the listeners your phone number and website address so that they know how to reach you for more information regarding your services.
- **Don't forget to remind the talk show host to give your phone number and website to the audience.** Remind him during a commercial break or before the next segment of the interview.
- **Tape your interviews.** This is a good way for you to critique and refine your interview skills. This will also give you samples that you can send to other talk show producers to improve your chances of being their guest.

Tips for After the Interview

- Send a simple thank you note to the show host for having you as a guest. This is common courtesy, but it also reinforces professionalism and your future spot as a returning guest.
- Request testimonials from show hosts. This greatly increases your credibility and opens doors for more interviews on other shows.
- Evaluate your interview/show success by the numbers of new clients and inquiries that are generated. The criteria of success is determined by how many people were motivated enough from hearing your information to pick up the phone or go to your website to inquire about your services or retain your services.
- Call the show producer or host and request a return appearance. Tell them about any new home care services you offer that will interest seniors and/or their particular

audience. (When they remember how compelling you were before, they will be happy to have you return!)

- Refine your interview over time. Expect to cover the same basic points in each interview, whether they are in the same order or not. The tapes of previous shows will help you plan and refine your talks.

CHAPTER FORTY-FIVE

Workshops, Trade Shows, Health and Job Fairs

If you want to hit a moving target, aim at where it's going to be, not at where it's at.

— Rene Bartos

You can also build your business by attending and participating in industry workshops, tradeshows, and public health and job fairs.

First, however, you must have a clear understanding of why you are participating or exhibiting in a particular event. Sit down and prepare a list of goals you want to achieve and prepare a summary of all the costs involved in this event. Will you get a return on your investment? If you know why you are attending and follow through on your goals, you can gain tremendously.

Why should you attend these events?

1. **Make sales**
   Since you are selling Home Care services and not products, you can use these events to get your company's name in front of prospective referral sources and/or

prospective clients. Be sure that you will be reaching these two target groups and be sure to have a method in place to get names, addresses and e-mails so you can follow up with letters and newsletters.

2. **Create or Support an Image**
   The quality and professionalism of your display unit, your staff and all the collateral material will all help to enhance the image you want to portray. Do not cut corners and attempt to slap something together at the last minute. First impressions are important.

3. **Introduce Your Services**
   These events give you an opportunity to be face to face with potential clients and referral sources. Use this opportunity to explain why your company is better than any other and why they should use your services.

4. **Be Compared to Your Competitors**
   This is an excellent opportunity to let people compare your company and services to those of your competitors.

5. **Market Research**
   Use these events as an opportunity to ask specific questions related to client needs or preferences. You can also obtain information about your competitors that will be valuable in planning and implementing future services and business strategies. Make sure you or your staff members prepare a report after the show, summarizing all the information you obtain.

6. **Publicity/Media**
   The media attend shows and Health Fairs looking for new trends and interesting stories for their readers. This can be a great opportunity to launch new services and get free publicity. Make sure you have a media kit to hand to the press if you get an opportunity to speak to them.

CHAPTER FORTY-SIX

Form Letters

We are what we believe we are.
We are what we repeatedly do.
Excellence, therefore, is not an act but a habit.
— Aristotle

You should have form letters available that you can customize. Form letters ensure that follow-up is done consistently throughout each office and each department.

Types of Form Letters to develop:

- Thank you letters to clients
- Thank you letters to referral sources (individual and company)
- Complaint responses
- Letters responding to inquiries
- Welcome letters for New Client Kits
- Letters reminding referral sources of other services that you offer

Thank You Letters and Cards

"Thank you" letters and cards create a positive feeling about your company. This is one of the least expensive ways to build loyalty, trust (and generate more referrals). Promptness matters, also. Send "Thank you" letters the day after you receive a referral.

You can use a form letter "Thank you," but make sure the letter is down--to-earth, genuine, sincere — *and personalized.*

Handwritten "Thank you" notes on letterhead cards will work as well. Having the form letter and cards pre-printed with your logo ensures uniformity and it also sends a message to your employees: We are an agency that puts emphasis on saying "Thank you."

THANK YOU: FOR A TESTIMONIAL FROM A REFERRING DOCTOR

Dear Dr. Johnson,

Thank you for sending the enthusiastic testimonial letter that I just received. Your kind response to my request for comments about (Our Home Care Agency) is greatly appreciated.

I am pleased that we have been able to provide home care services to many of your patients for the past five years, and that you have recommended our services to many of your colleagues and patients.

I appreciate your continued support. I promise to do everything in my power to maintain the high standards of quality and service you have learned to expect from us.

Again, thank you so much for the glowing testimonials.

Sincerely yours,

Name
Title

THANK YOU: FOR A TESTIMONIAL FROM A CLIENT

Dear Miss Cully,

Thank you for the testimonial I just received. Your praise of (Our Home Care Agency) is very gratifying and appreciated.

It is unusual for someone to take the time to express his or her satisfaction with services. It is people like you who make our special effort worthwhile.

I have passed your letter on to our supervisor and the caregivers, Sally Brown and Joyce Smith, who provided your care. We will be recognizing their special efforts in our next newsletter. I will make sure you receive a copy.

If you should require our services in the future, or if you know anyone else who requires help at home, I hope you will recommend our company.

Thank you again for the testimonial.

Cordially yours,

Name
Title

WELCOME LETTER

Dear Mrs. Johnson,

(Our Home Health Agency) thanks you for allowing us this opportunity to provide care and serve your nursing and personal needs.

Our staff are caring professionals dedicated to promoting the well being of our clients. We strive to demonstrate our belief in the dignity and individual rights of each individual.

If at any time you wish to discuss any aspect of your home care services, please do not hesitate to call our office and speak to a supervisor. He or she will immediately respond to your call and ensure that your concerns are attended to.

(Our Home Health Agency) stands behind our service guarantee. If for any reason you are not satisfied with our services, we will provide you with a full credit.

We look forward to assisting with your health care needs.

Sincerely yours,

Name
President

COMPLAINT RESPONSE LETTER

Dear Mrs. Johnson,

I have reviewed the situation you described in your letter of March 16, and I agree with you completely.

A mistake was made when you were not notified that your homemaker, Sally Smith, was ill and would not be able to make her visit to your home on March 10.

Instead of being sent another person without notification, you should have been told of Sally's illness and asked if you wished to have another homemaker fill in.

I apologize for the error and have discussed this with our staffing coordinators and supervisors to ensure this will be handled correctly in the future.

As a way of showing you how sorry we are for the error, we will pay for the services on March 10.

Again, please accept my apologies, and let me know if there is anything further I can do.

Sincerely yours,

Name
Title

APOLOGY FOR EMPLOYEE CONDUCT

Dear Mrs. Roberts,

Thank you for relating the unfortunate incident last week in which one of our staff was discourteous to you when you called our office.

I want to offer my personal apology and my promise that such inappropriate behavior will not occur again.

I have spoken with the employee about proper conduct and taken action to see that (his or her) attitude will change. I believe (he or she) realizes the gravity of (his or her) error.

Our staffs know the value of clients like you and are trained to handle your needs and problems efficiently and professionally. Unfortunately, mistakes do happen.

Please accept my apology. Your satisfaction and continued goodwill are our most important concerns.

Sincerely,

Name
Title

FOCUS GROUP LETTER

Dear Mrs. Johnson,

(Our Home Care Agency) would be pleased if you could participate in a focus group on community needs and resource planning which is being held on__________________.

The Health Care environment is rapidly changing, and no one knows that better than you. As a home care provider, (Our Home Health Care Company) is very interested in learning how these changes are affecting your patients and reshaping the needs of our community.

(Our Home Care Agency) has been providing Home Care Services in this community since 1995. Although we have established programs such as wound management, IV therapy, and support services for seniors, we are continuing to develop other programs and would value your input as we plan for the future.

We welcome your input and ask you to join your peers for this important discussion. Please call our office at 555–555–1212 by__________________if you would like to join us.

Best regards,

Name
Title

P.S. Should you be able to participate, we will be providing dinner and refreshments.

CHAPTER FORTY-SEVEN

How to Write Sales Letters... *That Sell!*

Write like you talk.

— Gary Halbert

The sales letter can be an extremely valuable marketing tool for your agency. Because the sales letter is perceived as person-to-person communication, it captures one of the key advantages over other marketing media in your mix — the voice of one person speaking to another. Our experience has been that a mailing containing a sales letter will perform better than a mailing without one.

Who do you send your sales letter to?

You should send your letter to referral sources — people whom you deem to be influential over those who are considering or are in immediate need of Home Care services. The following is a list of referral sources that will provide your agency with the most referrals.

- Case Managers (HMO's, Insurance Companies)
- Discharge Planners (Hospitals)

- Elderly (65–85 years of age)
- Children with elderly parents
- Trust Officers
- Administrators of assisted living facilities
- Physicians (General Practitioners)
- Funeral Home Directors

The best source for finding your list is the Standard Rate and Data Services (SRDS). This catalog/directory contains every commercially available mailing list, including source details, select prospects, and reference to list broker by category. This is where I recommend that you begin your search for the right list. Most main city public libraries have a current or year-old set of SRDS directories. Two great sources for prospect lists are:

1. Best Mailing Lists 1–800–NYC–BEST
2. Act One Mailing List Services 1–800–ACT–LIST

What are the Benefits of using a Sales Letter?

The sales letter can help your agency generate an immediate cash flow surge into your agency. How can it do this? A well-written sales letter, which contains a direct response message or an offer directed towards your prospect, compels the reader to take immediate action. There are very few marketing media that stimulate such prompt action from the prospect.

The sales letter provides your agency the opportunity to package its sales strategy and clone it! No matter how many sales people your agency has, it would be impossible to cold-call each and every potential prospect and deliver your sales presentation to them. There just isn't enough time to be able to physically accomplish this daunting task. But, by packaging your sales presentation into a letter, your agency can reach all of your prospects — not only once, but as many times as you need in order to make the sale.

Benefits of a Sales Letter

- 100% chance that your prospect will see your sales message!
- Person-to-person communication
- Increased response rate of direct-mail package
- Multiple sales presentations without face-to-face meetings
- Inexpensive
- Achieves a direct response from prospects
- Can include a promotion/sales offer
- Can test and/or change sales offer/promotion on demand
- Can include testimonials from happy clients

How do people read sales letters?

Writing interesting copy, having great testimonials and providing an irresistible sales/promotional offer isn't enough to create that perfect sales letter. You must be aware of *how* your prospect will read your letter so that you can learn to compose the layout of your sales letter for maximum readership.

People tend to scan a letter from top to bottom, looking for graphically emphasized words or phrases (headlines, subheadlines, captions, characters in uppercase, bold or italic type, underline, etc.). By using graphically emphasized words or phrases, your prospect will stop for a fraction of a second (according to some marketing experts, about two-tenths of a second) to read that one small part. This allows you to control what you want your prospect to focus on in your letter.

Spots on the letter that can grab your reader's attention:

- Headline above salutation
- Signature area
- Postscript (P.S.)
- First few paragraphs of your letter
- Highlighted copy
- Captions under an image
- Quotations and testimonials

Readers generally look at the signature area and glance at the P.S. before returning to the top of the first page. All of this takes just seconds. This holds true whether or not your letter is personalized with the recipient's name or has a generic greeting, like "Dear Discharge Planner." However, if your letter *is* personalized, the recipient will first look at his or her name, and *then* check the signature at the bottom of the letter. Then the recipient will resume the usual scanning pattern.

Do not underestimate the value of writing letters to prospective clients and referral sources. Good basic communication is good basic marketing. For example, if you write a letter to former clients, you will want to begin by thanking them for having used your services. Then tell them about the *new* services you have introduced, and any "special rates" or "discounts" you wish to promote. This is good communication, and it is very good marketing!

Your letter should:

- *Answer one basic question:* "What makes your agency so different that I, the reader, should do business with you?"
- *Be informative.* If someone is truly interested, they will want as much information as they can get so they can make a good decision.

- *Identify the key benefits your services will offer* to each of the individuals to whom you are writing.
- *Answer every objection they might have.* Send direct mail letters out at least three times. This generally doubles your response. To determine if direct mail is profitable, calculate the cost of mailing, including printing and postage. Calculate how much you profit from the mailing. If your profit is less than the cost to mail, that is when you stop mailing.

CHAPTER FORTY-EIGHT

Marketing Plan Think Sheets

"If you have built castles in the air, your work need not be lost. That is where they should be. Now put foundations under them."

— Henry David Thoreau

Your marketing plan is the heart of your company's business. To stay in business you have to constantly reach new clients and secure sales. This fillin-the-blank summary can help your agency develop its own marketing plan.

You may want to go through this exercise annually, every six months, every three months or even monthly, depending on the size, nature and maturity of your business.

Write Down Your Goals

One to six month goals (10)

1.______________________________

2.______________________________

3.______________________________

4.______________________________

5.______________________________

6.______________________________

7.______________________________

8.______________________________

9.______________________________

10.______________________________

Six to twelve month goals (10)

1.______________________________

2.______________________________

3.______________________________

4.______________________________

5.______________________________

6.______________________________

7.______________________________

8.______________________________

9.______________________________

10.______________________________

PART ONE – Develop Your Message!

STEP ONE: Features and Benefits

What are the *Features* and *Benefits* of your business, product, or service.

FEATURE	BENEFIT
1.____________________	1.____________________
2.____________________	2.____________________
3.____________________	3.____________________
4.____________________	4.____________________
5.____________________	5.____________________
6.____________________	6.____________________
7.____________________	7.____________________
8.____________________	8.____________________
9.____________________	9.____________________
10.___________________	10.___________________
11.___________________	11.___________________
12.___________________	12.___________________
13.___________________	13.___________________
14.___________________	14.___________________
15.___________________	15.___________________
16.___________________	16.___________________

STEP TWO: Your Unique Selling Proposition (USP)

____

____

____

____

____

____

Write 5 different headlines based on your USP:

1.____

2.____

3.____

4.____

5.____

STEP THREE: Develop Irresistible Offer(s)

Develop at least one irresistible offer compatible with your USP.

1.____

2.____

3.____

PART TWO: Your Service Niche

Explain the need of your client:

____

____

____

Explain why your services fulfill that need:

____

____

____

Explain why your service is the best:

____

____

____

Justify your price:

____

____

Give the reasons why prospects should call you today:

____

____

____

How can you build the prospect's interest in your service

1.________________________________

2.________________________________

3.________________________________

4.________________________________

5.________________________________

Develop Your Call to Action

1.________________________________

2.________________________________

3.________________________________

4.________________________________

5.________________________________

What do you want prospects to do?

1.________________________________

2.________________________________

3.________________________________

PART THREE: Your Target Market

What is your geographic target market:

____

____

____

What is your demographic target market:

____

____

____

Who are your referral sources:

1.______________________________________

2.______________________________________

3.______________________________________

4.______________________________________

5.______________________________________

6.______________________________________

7.______________________________________

8.______________________________________

9.______________________________________

10._____________________________________

11._____________________________________

12._____________________________________

13._____________________________________

14._____________________________________

15._____________________________________

PART FOUR: Your Credibility

List all the "TESTIMONIAL PROOF" you have:

Clients:

1.____

2.____

3.____

4.____

Celebrities:

1.____

2.____

3.____

List any other "PROOF" you have: i.e. articles, talkshows etc.

1.____

2.____

3.____

PART FIVE: Your Guarantee

Describe the guarantee(s) that you offer:

1.____

2.____

3.____

PART SIX: Your Image

Appearance of promotional material:

Brand-name identity:

Community Affairs:

Appearance of staff, vehicles, office:

PART SEVEN: Publicity

Charity/Non-profit ideas:

____

____

____

Positioning as an expert:

____

____

____

Creative promotions to media:

____

____

____

____

Talk shows:

____

____

____

____

Press kit:

____

____

____

PART EIGHT: Marketing Strategies

Inbound Telephone Procedures:

Outbound Telemarketing Strategies:

Coupon Ideas:

Direct Mail Campaign Ideas:

Trade Show, Health Fair Ideas:

____

____

____

____

____

Web Site Promotion Ideas:

____

____

____

____

____

Print Media Ideas: (Newspaper, Magazines)

____

____

____

____

____

Broadcast Media Ideas: (Television, Radio)

____

____

____

____

____

Signs/Billboard Ideas:

Referral Promotions:

Other:

PART NINE: Increasing client value

Service knowledge — Team training:

____

____

____

____

____

Special services offered:

____

____

____

____

____

New client admission procedure:

____

____

____

____

____

Complaint-Resolution process:

____

____

____

____

____

Client-Retention Plan:

____

____

____

____

____

Client-Promotion Ideas:

____

____

____

____

____

PART TEN: Your Marketing Budget

Marketing Strategy	Specifics	Frequency	Cost per Year
Image			
Collateral material			
Staff Uniforms			
Company vehicles			
Brochures/leaflets/fliers			
Print Media			
Newspaper			
Magazines			
Other			
Broadcast Media			
Television			
Radio			
Advertising Premiums			
Prospective clients			
Existing clients			
Direct Mail			
Web site			
Trade Shows			
Trade Show Display			
Signs/Billboards			
Public Relations/Publicity			
Networking (organizations)			
Other			
		TOTAL$	

PART TEN: Your Monthly Marketing Budget

Marketing Strategy	January	February	March	April	May	June	July	August	September	October	November	December	Total
Image													
Collateral material													
Staff Uniforms													
Company vehicles													
Brochures/leaflets/fliers													
Print Media													
Newspaper													
Magazines													
Other													
Broadcast Media													
Television													
Radio													
Advertising Premiums													
Prospective clients													
Existing clients													
Direct Mail													
Printing													
List Purchase													
Postage													
Mailing House													
Trade Shows													
Fees and setup													
Travel/Shipping													
Exhibits/signs													
Signs/Billboards													
Public Relations/Publicity													
Networking (organizations)													
Other													
												TOTAL $ ▶	

Referral-Boosting Home Care Sales and Marketing Tools

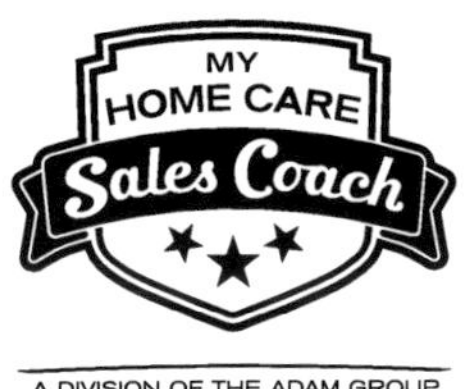

MyHomeCareSalesCoach.com

My Home Care Sales Coach is a members-only, resource-rich online community that gives you access to a wealth of easy-to-use and tried-and-proven tactics and strategies from home care sales and marketing experts. Membership includes access to PlayMaker CRM, a web-based, home care-specific contact management tool.

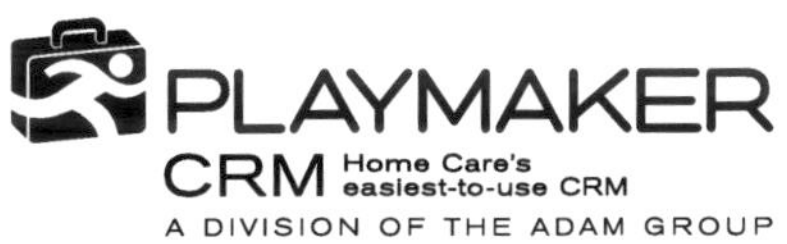

PlayMakerCRM.com

PlayMaker CRM is the first-of-its-kind contact management tool that is easy to use and specific to home care. It's a no software, no hardware, and no hassle solution to boosting your agency's sales and profits.

MAGNETIC MARKETING
for Home Care

MagneticMarketingForHomeCare.com

Magnetic Marketing for Home Care: How to Supercharge Your Referrals in Sixty Days or Less! Proven, easy-to-follow strategies to help agencies boost and retain referrals. Available in book and audio form.

Boot camps and additional sales and marketing coaching

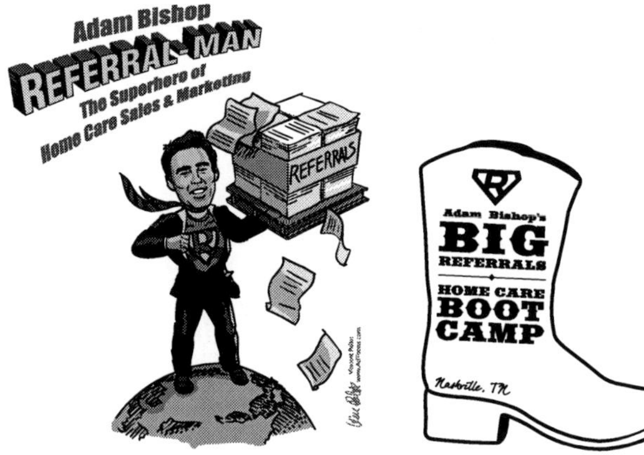

HomeCareReferralMan.com

Losing referrals to the competition? Reached a referral plateau? Not sure how to rev up the referral-boosting machine? Referral-Man to the rescue! He'll empower you with the knowledge and tools to send your referrals soaring.

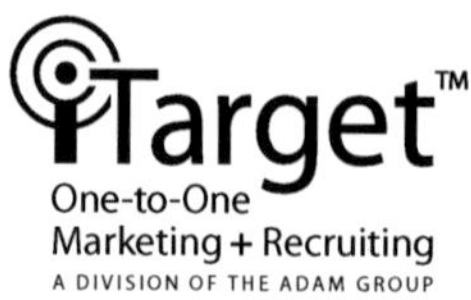

iTargetCampaigns.com

Zero in on your target audience with iTarget marketing and recruiting campaigns, which utilize the proven, revolutionary science of variable data. Whether you're marketing your services to referral sources or patients, or recruiting quality field staff, you'll create an interactive environment that guarantees results.